ILLNESS, RESILIENCE AND SPIRITUALITY

***

Edited by
Marguerite Guzmán Bouvard

For Griffen Saul
Founder
We Are Able

The man who says: I will conquer this illness and live a happy life, is already halfway through to victory.

Nelson Mandela

IN Publications

14 Lorraine Circle

Waban, MA 02468

Cover photo by Ariel V. Calver. Cover design by Jacques Bouvard.

Table of Contents

Introduction

We tend to think of illness as a physical problem, not realizing the emotional cost of severe physical and mental problems, and the need to change our lifestyles so that we no longer have the satisfaction of being able to accomplish what once seemed like easy tasks. For too many people who are living with serious illnesses, their daily lives are like climbing mountains, and unfortunately those efforts are often invisible.

Of greater significance, we often tend to overlook the creativity and courage of the seriously ill, how they rebuild their lives in different ways and contribute to their communities with new understanding and compassion. This is also true of those who are caring for loved ones with chronic conditions or who are dying, so the book is divided into two sections.

While the media carries stories of caring for elderly parents, not many people are aware of the heartache of caring for very ill children, including those who are dying. Caring for the dying in a society that is so afraid of death it is difficult to even have a conversation about what we now call "passing away," words that minimize a searing loss. It can be a lonely endeavor, but it is also possible to create a community of support, understanding and faith. Also, caring for a loved one who may be an older father or a grandfather or even a friend is a journey of sorrow and understanding. We grieve during an illness as we need to change our relationships with a transformed parent, child, or friend who may be suddenly a very different person.

One of the most powerful chapters in this book reveals how Carol Van de Woude, her family and her church cared tenderly and continually for her seven year old son, Steven, who became ill with leukemia. She created a world that would engage her son in learning, playing, and also read psalms with him. Members of her congregation were at their side, and Carol would continually give a list of prayers to them that would be said on his behalf. She even wrote a beautiful psalm herself when she knew that the end was near. Steven's twin sister was at his side when he was hospitalized for a month and his older sister, who was ten, went into the hospital to give her brother what he needed for a bone marrow transplant. Carol and her husband educated themselves about leukemia and shared their knowledge with their church. They also arranged for a teacher to come to the hospital and engage Steven who was a very bright child. The family stayed in the hospital with Steven when he was having chemotherapy and radiation and were available to him at all times, wearing masks and the proper clothes needed for his safety. While Carol and her family grieved, they created a community of faith and prayer, arranged for Steven not only to receive the best medical care, but to be engaged in education, amusing himself, and praying. The words Carol heard during her trials remind us of the connection between this world and eternity, *Steven will be okay but you need to be comforted.*

Christina Chiu's chapter about living with a little son who has VACTERL, (vertebral, anal, cardiac, tracheal, esophageal and renal) is a story of courage, despair and joy. She faced accompanying her son Tyler through six surgeries as well as seeing a gastroenterologist, and home visits from occupational therapists, physical therapists, and nutritional consultants. Also, she needs to give him a daily colostomy because her son's bowels don't work. She lives with fatigue, frustration, sorrow, but also with joy because of her deep love for her son. In the early years of coping with her son's physical problems she asked herself why this was happening to her tiny son, and to her. She told herself that Buddha's lesson about life as suffering, didn't respond to her situation. Also, she does not have the support she needs through her grueling days. Her parents express no interest and her husband is more than busy with his job. But this young woman has achieved great wisdom. Her support is her Buddhist faith that has taught her that without suffering we cannot experience true joy. Through her difficult journey, she has acquired strength, extraordinary coping skills, and deep compassion for her son. In the midst of all this hard work of adjusting to a difficult situation, Christina Chiu was able to write an extraordinary book of short stories as well as a novel, revealing that everything is possible regardless of the circumstances.

Jean Colgan Gould's chapter, We Are On the Floor Talking, is both a touching love story, and the way a loving wife accompanies her husband through illness and death. It is a series of conversations that reveals their similarities, and their differences, conversations they have had throughout the years of their marriage, and the depth of understanding between them. What makes this chapter so wonderful is that it reveals dying as another way of living well, while the couple continues their daily life together and as the husband keeps thinking about work, politics and more. Throughout his bout with lymphoma and the effects of his heart attack, he is deeply engaged with the world and his opinions. Death appears briefly during conversations about their intertwined lives and more, "Give everything away to the poor," Irving comments in the middle of a conversation about the wall paper. There is humor in this chapter as well. Since Irving is Jewish and Jean is Catholic, they attend a service at a chapel in the Brandeis University campus. It is held by a Catholic priest who was defrocked by the Boston Archdiocese for speaking out against sexual abuse of children by priests. His opening statement is highly unusual as he welcomes, "Catholics, non-Catholics, gay or straight," and "our Jewish and Muslim sisters and brothers." This chapter defies our views of death and celebrates the love that never dies.

Nancy Gerber's chapter on her father's stroke is deeply moving and wide ranging. We read about how her father changed from a busy man who was head of the family, a loving husband, father and grandfather, into an unrecognizable person who lay quietly in a hospital and nursing homes, a man who played tennis, who was gregarious and had many friends and loved his life. When he had his first stroke, he was 73 and still working, and looking forward to traveling with his wife. Nancy watched him ebb away unable to talk, walk or move. Her feelings included guilt and a never ending grief. Her mother, brother and herself spent hours sitting by his bed. He was in a hospital and in acute and sub-acute care and then in a nursing home. Nancy's Jewish faith meant so much to her, and to her father, yet she wrote, "there is no language for such a loss, no prayers or rituals for the death of someone who hasn't died." She was with him while he died and asked him to say her name and if he understood her, and he did both.

Losing a cherished friend who shares your passions and also helps you through some difficult moments in your life is heart breaking. Pierre Bouvard and Brad Saul were both deeply involved with radio even when they were students at Northwestern University. They lived and talked radio for long hours, and immersed themselves in that field in many different ways while getting through their courses. They remained very close friends after their graduation, were in constant touch and even went on a vacation to Europe together. They were at each other's weddings, and celebrated the birth of their children. Brad helped Pierre through some difficult decisions about his work and a relationship that didn't bode well before he met the wonderful woman he married. When Brad became ill with multiple sclerosis at the age of 30, he continued his work in radio, and because of his physical limitations came up with new visions for that field and read voraciously about his illness. He created the Radio Center for People With Disabilities to recruit, train and place people with disabilities into radio stations, and inspired a taxi company to create a special service for the disabled. When he and his wife Debbie decided on palliative care because he was close to death, Pierre flew down to be at his side. He called Brad's friends to be with him as well and they dropped everything and came immediately, so Brad was surrounded with love. Pierre remembers giving him a hug before he left. When Brad died three days later, Pierre and his wife Mary flew down to participate in the services at Brad's synagogue, and to take part in the Shiva. Losing such a close friend is like losing a brother, but with time Pierre celebrates his memories of such a remarkable person as Brad.

Tara Coyote reveals that a person who is struggling with third stage cancer can also reach out and help people suffering with grief. We rarely view seriously ill people as able to offer help and enlarge their lives. Tara witnessed cancer first hand by caring for her two closest friends and witnessing the death of her best friend. Shortly after, she was diagnosed with cancer herself. Having seen the side effects of chemotherapy and radiation, and her friend die as a 65 pound skeleton, she decided to heal herself in an unusual way. She changed her diet, and she periodically takes RGCC tests that measure the tumor cells circulating in the blood, a practice used in other countries but not in the U.S. She practices Kundalini Yoga where she has profound spiritual experiences, and an understanding that even though the body dies, the spirit remains alive. During these exercises she felt a profound peace and love. Despite living with her illness she created a horse farm, the Wind Horse Sanctuary where she gave lessons on healing from grief because she knows how we can communicate with horses in a nonverbal language that calms our emotions. In fact veterans from the wars in Iraq and Afghanistan who are suffering from PTSD (Post Traumatic Stress Disorder) are given dogs by a non-profit organization that trains service dogs, K9s for Warriors.[1] A veteran who is overwhelmed with anger, and with a traumatic brain injury, can step outside of a room with his dog that is able to share his emotions.

Sister Pamela Smith pairs her serious illness, "brittle diabetes" with her growing spiritual awareness and her decision to join the community of The Sisters of Saint Cyril and Methodius, named after two Greek priests who translated the bible into Cyrillic for Slavic peoples in Eastern Europe. She feels close to Saint Cyril because one of her goals became translating the gospel to her contemporaries, young people and adults, people who go to mass and who never attend mass. Her type of diabetes, a life threatening disease that requires regular blood tests, urine tests, medications, and creates dizziness and visual problems when her blood sugar is low, plus several bouts in the emergency room, did not prevent her from working towards her Ph.D; teaching writing, and human service, that are her passions. Sister Pamela has publicized her respect for different religions, Zen, Islam and Judaism, has offered reflections on African saints at a Black Heritage Month day of prayer, and conducted a short retreat at an eco-spiritual center hosting a group of sisters from Canada, Australia, Kenya, and the U.S. But the work which has touched her the most has been her meetings with homeless men. She writes that there is a brokenness living with her chronic illness, and waking up to her fragility made her see and empathize with someone else's brokenness, to see the spirit of God everywhere and in everyone.

Neil Orts is a writer and has devoted his life to creating unusual art performances that at times are available not only to audiences but also to passersby when they take place before a very large window. He intertwined his medical care with creating his performances, as well as his spirituality, for he insists that his art projects are his primary concern. His journey through illness was long, complicated and very trying. A physician had found a large mass on his pancreas that might have been cancerous. Neil knew a lot about cancer since when he had attended seminary, he did a summer of Clinical Pastoral Education on a cancer floor in a hospital. Also both of his parents died of cancer. When the mass was removed Neil spent some difficult times in the hospital and afterwards, wondering if was going to survive. Yet throughout this difficult period he was deeply involved in producing performances such as a Light and Shadow performance that reflected his situation. He also put on a one man show with a special covering on his body and invited the audience to make a mark on the part of his body where a person was experiencing pain. As always he turned to his spiritual leaders throughout his days. Fortunately, the mass was cancer free yet led to diabetes. He turned continually to the Desert Fathers and Mothers, the Abbas and Ammas, particularly Abba Macarius, were with him, and not only kept him focused on God's mercy, but helped him laugh through it all. Having faced the possibility of death, he never lost his sense of humor.

Victoria's Molta's life has been a remarkable journey through family problems, mental illness, to a life of love, compassion and activism. She writes about a difficult and lonely childhood, about her father who was alcoholic, mentally disturbed and who frightened her with his stories and his behavior. Her mother leaned on her when she was young, using her as a source of support after arguments with her father. But it was her great-grandmother who deeply influenced her. She was an artist who divorced a difficult husband at a time when this was an unusual step for a woman. Also, she was deeply religious and very loving with Victoria. The time she spent with her great-grandmother influenced her life profoundly. She had a mental breakdown when she was twenty four years old and was diagnosed with bipolar disorder. Some years later she received a diagnosis of schizoaffective disorder, a psychotic disorder that includes recurring episodes of mood changes as well as a loss of contact with reality. Her illness brought her to mental hospitals where she stayed for months and received treatments that were often less than helpful. But she had the inner strength to leave these situations and a deep faith that she had felt since she was a child. She left a hospital where she had been for three months that wanted to transfer her to a mental institution, deciding to see another psychiatrist who helped her not to be cured, but to recover. Despite her difficult life, Victoria had a strong sense of independence and prayed continually for courage, for she knew that her spirit was stronger than her illness. For some years she lived in a half way house where she met a man she fell in love with. They have been married for twenty four years, living in their own home. She now works in the Connecticut mental health movement as an advocate and a counselor, speaks to audiences about her recovery, and lobbies her legislators for housing for people with mental illnesses. These are just a few of her many incredible efforts to create much needed support.

Wendy Devitt is yet another heroine who dealt with vision problems on an ongoing basis. She was born with congenital cataracts and had surgery to remove them when she was very young. In her early years, she pretended that she could see well although the glare of sunlight through a window prevented her from seeing the black board in her classroom, and it took her a long time to do her homework. Also, she could see better in one eye than another which furthered her difficulties, but she continued to pursue her life as if nothing was wrong. In high school she even drove to events with her friends at night, because she wanted to spend time with them. She wanted to have a normal life and didn't realize the importance of seeing well. When she was eighteen, she developed glaucoma and went to see a specialist for a number of tests. She was given eyedrops to lower the pressure in her eyes and then pills when the eye drops stopped helping to alleviate her condition. But she is a person who never gives up and attended Florida State University and then moved to New York City where she received a degree. She then applied for a job to the Perkins School for the Blind in Boston and was accepted. At this time she began taking Yoga classes with some of her colleagues that would change her life. She bought a book, Light on Yoga, by BSK Iyengar and found ways of relaxing and allowing herself to feel the emotions about her eyesight that were healing. She also decided to move to New York City and was accepted with a full scholarship at Columbia University Teachers College where she received a Master of Arts that would enhance her knowledge of teaching visually impaired children. In 2016 she spent the summer in India working with Geeta Iyengar on Yoga. She knew that she was on an ongoing journey learning acceptance and compassion. While she was periodically having surgery throughout her life, she had discovered the joy of not only teaching, but helping visually impaired primary school students and teens learn yoga.

People who remember the war in Vietnam, think of the divisiveness it sparked in our country and the demonstrations against it. Fortunately Ken Burns has produced a wonderful documentary of the war in Vietnam, But few people are aware of how our soldiers who fought in that war have suffered. Post Traumatic Stress Disorder has entered our thoughts for the soldiers who served in Iraq and Afghanistan, although too many people do not know about how it has affected our veterans from Vietnam. It means nightmares, inability to sleep, strong reactions to noises, trouble keeping a marriage together and more. Memories of death and destruction have become part of our Vietnam veterans' lives. Preston H. Hood's chapter is a powerful story of what our veterans have endured. He recalls jumping out of a helicopter and running to a fellow soldier who committed suicide only to see his brains blown out trying to save him. His lungs and heart were affected by the Agent Orange we sprayed to kill the foliage if enemies were near. Preston also writes about his heart condition which is intertwined with his stories about the war, and how his own son's suicide affected him and his family. This chapter is an unusual and remarkable translation of PTSD for people who have never experienced it. Telling the truth is very powerful and courageous. Not many people are able to share this kind of pain in their lives. Yet Preston H. Hood is a very gifted and sensitive writer who reveals the complexity of living with two lives; war and stateside where he is surrounded by people who have had the good fortune of living with only one life. He practices and teaches Yoga Nidra, which helps him to relax and heal.

Maria Bernardi's chapter is unusual because it is written in two sections, the first is about coming down with three chronic illnesses in the midst of a busy life as a professor and a volunteer involved in sponsoring and supporting refugees, and writing books. Suddenly, her life fell apart since she had to quit her job, and had insufficient energy to pursue her volunteer work. Living with Interstitial Cystitis, (IC), fibromyalgia and Chronic Fatigue seemed to place her on another planet. However, when she was in the first stages of IC, she was able to travel to a conference of Cherokee women in Tahlequah Oklahoma where she met Awiakta, who became a close friend and opened her up to a new way of life that was intensely spiritual. It remained with her as a guide that would give her inner strength throughout her life. Eventually, she also found help for IC, and read a book about fibromyalgia that was very useful. However many years later she had four very serious medical malpractices, one was a prescription that caused her to pass out on the bathroom floor, become unconscious and hemorrhage in her brain, causing a traumatic brain injury. Yet another physician prescribed an overdose of Xanax that addicted her and eventually removed her ability to sleep. In fact, NPR published an article in April, 2016 [2] that was written by researchers at the John Hopkins School of Medicine revealing that the third cause of death in the United States after Heart Disease and Cancer was medical malpractice. The lead author of the research team wrote an open letter to the Center for Disease Control and Prevention to immediately add medical errors to its annual list reporting the top causes of death.[3] Maria received help from a very loving family. Her husband, who accompanied her through these trials, her daughter who bought her a mini laptop to take notes since she had lost her short term memory as a result of her brain injury, her niece who edited her books and her granddaughter who sent her a teddy bear with so much love. Once again, Maria is not only writing books, but reaching out to help people in need such as a Syrian refugee who was suffering with PTSD (Post Traumatic Stress Disorder), and she has learned how to count her blessings.

This book is a revelation of the many possibilities in difficult lives; flexibility, moving on to new ways of living, continuing to be productive, and sharing one's talents with others who are suffering. When we think of strength, we may consider ambition, success, or physical prowess. However there are the important traits of inner strength, faith, and compassion.

NOTES

1. Emilie Le Beau Lucchesi. "When Animals Sense and Influence our Feelings." *International New York Times.* 6/9/17.

2. Marshall Allen, NPR, 4/16/16.

3. Ibid.

Prayers Through Illness and Loss
by Carol Van Der Woude

After a two-week period of nagging leg pains, my son developed severe bone pain. Our pediatrician referred us to Children's Memorial Hospital. From the admitting office we were directed to a hospital room. I gasped when I read the sign on the unit, 7 West Oncology. Steven was admitted to the cancer unit, and I was frightened. I didn't know it then, but I was at the beginning of a spiritual journey. Prayer became increasingly important.

During that first night at the hospital, I wept in the parents' lounge. The only prayer I could utter came with a river of tears. "O Lord, not Steven. Not this child. This is not what I expected for my son. Not this." I felt like I had been punched in the gut.

The next morning we were called into a conference room. A hematologist told us that the blood tests confirmed that Steven had leukemia. We had two days to absorb Steven's diagnosis while his body was being prepared for chemotherapy.

On Monday morning the battle for Steven's life began with a tornado of activity. Steven endured bone marrow aspiration, a spinal tap and a blood transfusion. A surgeon came to examine Steven and discuss placement of a central line catheter for the purpose of chemotherapy.

The urgency of the procedures was not lost on Steven. He asked me, "How long am I going to be sick?" He waited for a response, and as I groped for an answer he asked, "How long am I going to be in the hospital?"

My mind was full of questions. I didn't know how to answer. Finally I said, "I don't know."

"You know! You have to know!" Steven screamed. He wanted assurance that his father and I had control of this situation. We were his parents, we were supposed to know.

My heart was breaking. I couldn't stop tears from coming to my eyes. I tried to explain that leukemia is a serious illness. "We have to take this one step at a time. God knows about this and we have to trust Him to help us." I held his hands in mine.

My knowledge of God directed me to trust Him. Everything that I had learned about God, through Bible study and a personal relationship with Jesus, gave me faith to believe in God's goodness.

I realized that my son needed to turn to God, so I prayed with him. A few days later Steven and I read Isaiah 40:26-31. The passage begins, "Lift up your eyes on high and see who created these? He who brings out their host by number, calling them all by name . . ." We talked about God creating the heavens and the stars. Together Steven and I wrote out the full passage in booklet form. Steven drew pictures and pasted magazine pictures on the pages to illustrate the verses. I encouraged him to memorize this passage of scripture.

My husband, Dan, and I focused on learning as much as we could about leukemia. We studied the high-risk treatment protocol that Steven was placed on. I wrote a letter for our church with specific prayer requests.

"As Dan and I struggle to cope with Steven's diagnosis, we are gathering information about leukemia. During the past ten years tremendous progress has been made in the area of childhood leukemia. Of children that have acute lymphocytic leukemia, 90% go into remission, 50% are still in remission after five years. (We did not know at the time that Steven had a more aggressive form of leukemia).

Steven is on a protocol of treatment that is based on a national computer database. According to Steven's doctor, the outlook is positive and hopeful.

Understanding the disease process relieves some of our fears and also helps us pray more specifically for Steven. Acute lymphocytic leukemia begins in the bone marrow. Bone marrow is a fluid like material located in the center of bones. Bone marrow is responsible for the production of red blood cells, white blood cells and platelets. For some unknown reason the bone marrow begins to malfunction.

Instead of producing normal cells it begins producing thousands of baby white cells. The baby cells (blasts) do not carry out a function and instead crowd out red blood cells and platelets. Eventually the blasts spill over into the bloodstream, causing anemia, problems with bruising and bleeding, and decreasing the body's ability to fight infection.

The goal of chemotherapy (medication which destroys rapidly growing cells) is to destroy all of the leukemic blasts. Unfortunately the medication can also destroy some of the red blood cells and platelets. Blood or platelet transfusions may be necessary. As the blasts are destroyed the number of normal white cells dips quite low and infections can become dangerous because there are not enough white cells to fight infection.

Another goal of treatment is to prevent the spread of leukemia cells to other parts of the body. For that reason medication is injected into the spinal fluid and radiation therapy is indicated. These treatments will reach any "hiding" blasts.

We are praising God that no leukemia cells have been found in Steven's spinal fluid. He is tolerating the initial phase of chemotherapy very well. After one week in the hospital he was able to come home and is being treated on an outpatient basis. Steven is eating well and spends a lot of time working on our computer. Please pray for the following concerns:

1. Since the beginning of this illness Steven has had pain and tenderness in his legs. The tenderness has improved greatly. He is able to stand and take a few steps but is not walking much. Pray that he will regain strength in his legs.

2. As a part of treatment Steven requires blood transfusions. We are praising God that we have found some A, CMV negative blood donors. In the event that

*blood must be given from the blood bank, pray that the
blood will be free of the AIDS virus.*

*3. As we continue through chemotherapy, pray that
Steven will experience minimal side effects.*

*4. Pray that Steven's bone marrow will produce
normal white cells.*

5. Pray that Steven will remain free of infection."

My life became focused on Steven's care. We were blessed to
have friends bring us meals during the days that were filled with
medical treatments. We were blessed to have neighbors that were
ready to pray with us. Sometimes we met on the driveway and
joined hands to pray.

The summer went by, and in the fall Steven was in remission.
He was due to enter first grade along with his twin sister. He still
had a central line catheter, but he was given the permission to
attend half days of school.

The nurse clinician at Children's Memorial Hospital and the
school nurse worked with me to plan for Steven's participation.
The greatest concerns were exposure to infection and accidental
harm to the central line catheter in Steven's chest. The school
nurse taught Steven's classmates and their parents about the
importance of hand washing. We agreed that it would be helpful if
I made myself available if any problems arose with the central
line.

My mornings were free so I took little projects with me to the
elementary school. I sat in the teachers' lounge while Steven was
in class and got to know the staff at the school. Steven's twin sister
was in a different classroom, but she was steadfast in protecting
him.

It touched my heart to see her march up to a boy that was
teasing Steven because of his hair loss due to chemotherapy. She
told him to leave her brother alone, and he stopped.

Summer came. It was one year since Steven's diagnosis. At
his clinic appointment I learned that the cancer cells were back. He
looked healthy, but his blood counts showed that he had relapsed. I

was shaken. Steven was given an immediate dose of chemotherapy, and I called a dear friend and asked her to pray for us. My husband Dan was out of town. I hated to give him this news over the phone.

We were entering a new phase. The doctor said a bone marrow transplant might save Steven's life. We would need to go to a medical center that performed bone marrow transplant. Should we take this next step? Where should we go?

We began to do research but we also asked for prayer from our church. I felt wooden and numb as I provided the facts for our church friends. During this period of searching, Dan and I visited our pastor and his wife. We requested that the laying on of hands with prayers for healing be done for Steven. Our pastor had never done this before, but he believed that it was biblical. He called a meeting with the elders of the church and the bone marrow transplant procedure was discussed.

We found out that Steven's older sister Sara was a complete match for bone marrow transplant. Specific factors in her blood matched Steven's, making transplant possible. I was grateful and anxious at the same time.

A week later the pastor, elders and deacons came to our home. Dan had explained to Steven the type of prayer that was going to take place. Each man prayed for Steven and rubbed oil on his forehead. Steven was quiet and accepting. He appeared encouraged.

We left our home community and traveled to the Fred Hutchinson Cancer Treatment Center (FHCTC) in Seattle as a family. After Steven and Sara had initial tests we waited for a bed to open up. We used the time as if we were on vacation.

We were fortunate to arrive in Seattle in late July, the best time to go to this maritime city. Most of the year Seattle has overcast skies but instead of the rain and clouds, we enjoyed summer sunshine. The air was fresh and vibrant with the mist from the nearby ocean.

As a family we visited picturesque places within driving distance. We went to Mt. Rainier National Park. The kids were at a good age to enjoy the forests, meadows and waterfalls along with the spectacular view of Mt. Rainier. Sara was ten years old. Julia and Steven were seven years old.

We took a picture of Sara, Steven and Julia standing in a little circle of ground surrounded by huge trees. We tried to capture the joy and wonder in Steven's brown eyes. We discovered trees with large hollows and climbed on fallen trees. The mountain air was cool and fresh, invigorating. Steven wrote about this adventure in a scrapbook, "When we looked at the trees some of them looked like houses."

On another day we took a boat ride across Elliot bay to Blake Island. Blake Island was the site of an ancient Indian campground. We visited Tillicum village where Northwest Indians demonstrated aspects of their culture, including colorful costumes, brightly painted masks and totem poles. We enjoyed a salmon dinner as the Indians performed native dances.

We were fascinated by the traditional preparation of the salmon. The big salmon fillets were fastened to wooden poles and cooked over huge fire pits. Steven said that it was the best salmon that he had ever tasted.

Perhaps it was the prayers being offered for us that gave us the peace of mind to enjoy our new surroundings. We had a special family vacation in a beautiful setting.

Steven was admitted to the Cancer Research Center on August 23rd. We had a long conference with the medical team. We were told that Steven's leukemia was complicated by a high-risk marker, the Philadelphia chromosome. They gave him a 25% chance of survival with bone marrow transplant.

The severity of Steven's situation was clear. I realized that trusting God was not something that I had achieved. Trust was a continuing process that needed to be renewed each day.

Steven was scheduled to receive high doses of chemotherapy, plus four days of radiation therapy, to prepare for the infusion of bone marrow from his sister. His private room was divided into two sections. The divider consisted of a wall halfway up. The upper half was a clear plastic drape that we could see through.

His living space was enclosed in a sterile laminar airflow system. The outer section of the room was equipped with a cot where Dan or I could spend the night. Steven would remain in his sterile space throughout transplant and recovery. Whenever caregivers or family members entered the sterile compartment they had to gown and glove.

Each family member was a participant in Steven's care. Dan managed to hook up a computer system for Steven to work on while he was confined. Sara was prepared to be the bone marrow donor. Julia dressed up in the sterile gown, gloves and mask to enter Steven's room and entertain him with games.

I wrote a prayer letter for our church with these requests:

> *"1. During the time that chemotherapy and radiation are given, pray that God will use these treatments to get rid of all cancer cells. Pray also that God will protect Steven's healthy cells, especially brain, liver and lungs.*
>
> *2. Pray that our doctors will be given wisdom and guidance from God.*
>
> *3. Pray for continued good communication lines with the medical staff.*
>
> *4. Pray that all blood products that are given to Steven will be protected from infective agents.*
>
> *5. Pray that both Sara and Steven will experience God's care and comfort as they are hospitalized."*

After Steven had a urinary catheter placed he had bladder spasms through the night. I gowned and gloved to enter his space and give comfort. On other nights he had episodes of diarrhea, probably due to the antibiotics he was getting as prophylaxis. Dan and I took turns spending the night next to his sterile room, ready to gown and glove if Steven needed help.

As the day for bone marrow transfusion approached, I was with Steven, assisting him with a change of hospital gown. As I lifted the gown I accidentally tugged on his central line catheter and Steven screamed. I called the nurse and she called a resident doctor. On examination, part of the cuff seemed to have moved and the site was tender. The resident doctor said, "We are too close to transplant to do anything. This will have to work."

Steven and I prayed together. Later, outside of his room I was tormented with fears. I was laying out my fear before God in prayer. I was restless. Words came to me—words that did not originate from me. *Steven will be okay, but you need to be comforted.* It was such an unusual experience that the words were burned into my memory. In the following days I wrote this psalm for Steven.

> *"O Lord God,*
> *You created Steven*
> *just as you created the birds,*
> *the flowers and the stars.*
> *When Steven became ill*
> *You strengthened him.*
> *You were with him through*
> *all of the painful tests.*
> *You restored him*
> *And he was protected.*
> *Now the cancer has come back.*
> *We are in agony.*
> *The next test is harder than*
> *all the others.*
> *Bone marrow transplant with*
> *Dangers and side effects are before us.*
> *We are here in Seattle.*
> *We pray that we won't be overwhelmed with fear.*
> *Show us more about Yourself.*
> *We want to know you.*
> *You do love us.*
> *Lord, we trust you*
> *to continue to care for Steven.*
> *And as you care for him,*

let us know you better.
You love us all."

For bone marrow donation, Sara was admitted to the neighboring hospital. She received anesthesia as marrow was aspirated from her hips. She was sore for a couple days, but hopeful that her marrow would help Steven live.

The bone marrow was rushed over by messenger to be infused like a blood transfusion into Steven. Later that day Sara was transported by wheelchair to Steven's room for a visit. She came through a tunnel that connected the neighboring hospital to the Cancer Research Center.

Over the following days the transplant seemed to be successful. Fever and rash were signs of graft versus host disease, the new marrow was growing and Steven's body was reacting. Medications were given to relieve his symptoms.

Steven remained in the hospital for more than a month. During this time the girls attended the Hutch School that was for cancer patients and their siblings. They were introduced to a cooperative game, Save the Whales. The players work together to save endangered whales from environmental hazards and the pirate ship. The goal of the game is to get each whales into a safe haven. Eventually Steven and I played this game too.

When Steven was discharged from the hospital Dan and the girls went home. Our apartment was small and we needed to decrease the chance of infection. On October 16th I wrote this letter to our friends.

"The Lord is my strength and my shield; in him my heart trusts, and I am helped. My heart exults and with my song I give thanks to him. The Lord is the strength of his people." Psalm 28:7-8

This verse holds a promise that we have clung to. One Christian friend did a word study on the word, shield. She gave us a list of verses in the Psalms that have encouraged and comforted us. Steven has enjoyed reading and learning verses from the Psalms. As we studied the verses we talked about David's years in the wilderness and in Philistine territory, and God's care for David. Give thanks with us because Steven is out of the hospital! We have completed the most difficult part of treatment and the Lord has watched over us.

Psalm 32: 8-11 is also a comfort. This passage begins, "I will instruct you and teach you in the way you should go; I will counsel you with my eye upon you." Through the prayers of many, and through the ministry of our church, God has shown us the way in the many decisions surrounding Steven's treatment. Our doctors have been able to make recommendations for us but have also acknowledged their limitations. Our trust is in God.

During the next two months Steven and I will be staying in Seattle while Steven receives follow-up treatment. Steven is taking medication to control the graft versus host reaction, to maintain his body minerals and to maintain a normal blood pressure. Three times a week he has blood tests, once a week a physical exam, a chest x-ray and a nutritional counseling meeting. Twice a week he is tutored. We keep a busy schedule.

Dan, Sara and Julia are at home in Chicago. They have returned to school and work routines. We are grateful to our neighbors who have been taking care of our home while we were gone. My sister and the grandparents will all be involved in keeping our household running over the next two months.

One Plus One, Mother of Twins, our Home Owners Association, and elementary school have all raised funds to meet our medical, travel and living expenses. We have been free of financial stress and have been able to focus on getting well.

We ask that God will bless each of you as you pray for Steven's continued recovery. Staying free of infection and being able to reduce medication levels are important goals for Steven. Thank-you for your support."

The time that Steven and I had together during these two months of outpatient care was a gift. We were busy with appointments, but on occasion we went to the public library during hours that had less traffic. Steven wore a mask, and we went out on the second floor open porch. Steven brought some crackers to feed the pigeons. It was a moment of joy.

At night we took a telescope outside to look at the moon. Steven had an insatiable curiosity. We read books. We visited a card shop and read the funny cards out loud. We watched the World Series together.

At the final medical conference before Steven was released to go home, the hematologists noticed some signs that were troubling. They made some cautionary statements, but released us to go home for Christmas. A couple of paragraphs from our Christmas letter to friends reflected the joy.

> *"It has been a pleasure to receive Christmas cards and notes. One of the blessings of Christmas is to hear from those that are dear to us. Our joy this holiday season has been great, because after months of separation we are once again together as a family .*

> *Recovery from bone marrow transplant is a slow process, requiring careful medical monitoring. By day 100 post transplant most problems that can occur have shown up. So in December Steven and I came home with plans for his care here. We now go back to Children's Memorial Hospital once a week for blood tests and physical exam. Home is more wonderful than ever before.*

> *Dan and I are catching up on our rest now. The past months have been exhausting. We are well and most thankful for God's care."*

When we returned to clinic visits at Children's Memorial Hospital, the transition from FHCRC was difficult. Steven was now receiving a long list of medications. His care was complex and the clinic was busy. Within three weeks his blood counts showed that he had relapsed.

On January 22nd Steven developed a high fever and was admitted to the hospital. After a couple days of intravenous fluids and antibiotics Steven was stabilized. But our doctor did something that stunned us. While standing at Steven's bedside he told us (and Steven) that all hope was gone. I shuddered. Steven needed some hope for the days ahead.

We were released from the hospital and referred to a home care agency. Soon we realized that the home care nurse was not informed of all the medications that Steven had been prescribed after his transplant. We were concerned about stopping some medications suddenly. Our communication with our doctor at the clinic was frustrating. We prayed for direction.

A pediatric hematologist from the Sloan-Kettering Cancer Center in New York was now head of a pediatric cancer unit at a nearby hospital. We called him and told him our story. He agreed to see Steven, but reserved his decision to take on his care until after our appointment. Steven made an impression. This doctor agreed to coordinate his care. He gave thorough instructions to the home care agency, and arranged for blood transfusions and one more round of chemotherapy.

We agreed on a plan of care that allowed Steven to be cared for at home. The home care nurse came out for the transfusions and periodic checks. Dan and I became Steven's caregivers. Dan learned how to manage intravenous fluids and made suggestions for the equipment we were using. When Steven no longer had the appetite to eat sufficiently, he received intravenous fluids as nourishment. The fluids ran at night while Steven slept.

Many nights I sat outside Steven's bedroom door while the intravenous fluid was running. Even though I was a nurse, I didn't feel adequately prepared to provide support for my dying child. My prayers became questions.

I had discovered novels written by George MacDonald, a Scottish pastor. MacDonald was a contemporary of Charles Dickens. He was acquainted with the death of family members, and his stories dealt with death in a practical and prayerful way. He gave me insight into how to walk alongside Steven.

On the days that Steven was feeling well enough he had a tutor that had been arranged by our elementary school. The first time Miss L. came to our home, she greeted Steven with enthusiasm and asked to have a workplace separate from household activities. She brought projects and stimulated Steven's interest. I heard them talking and laughing together.

When Steven relapsed I was afraid to tell her. I wanted Steven to be treated normally without sympathy or sadness. I did not want the joy of their time together to change. The problem was that Steven's good days became unpredictable. I had to cancel several tutoring times because Steven was sick.

Miss L. confronted me. "I need to know what is going on. Please tell me."

With some misgiving I told her that Steven had relapsed again. We didn't know how much longer he would be with us. With the air cleared Miss L. drew a breath and responded. "Just let me know. We will continue our sessions when Steven wants to."

I had underestimated Miss L. She focused on Steven's gifts and talents. They began writing their own version of the children's story, Goldilocks. Steven looked forward to the tutoring sessions.

On other days, leaders from our church's club for children (Awana) visited and helped Steven with Bible verses. He was listening to Bible verses on tape, memorizing and discussing them. My heart was touched when he talked about these verses.

> _"Behold the dwelling place of God is with man. He will dwell with them, and they will be his people, and God himself will be with them as their God. He will wipe away every tear from their eyes, and death shall be no more, neither shall there be mourning, nor crying, nor pain anymore, for the former things have passed away."_
> _Revelation 21: 3-4_

Evenings were for family time. Often friends brought us meals. After dinner we played family games, and Steven pushed past fatigue to participate.

On March 11th our family attended a regional Awana club event. Steven carried the flag for the opening ceremonies. Only people from our church were aware of Steven's illness. At the end of the day Steven wrote is his diary. *"Awana stands for approved workmen are not ashamed."*

On April 22nd Steven's body was failing. He was receiving a continuous morphine drip for pain control. In the morning our pastor and his wife visited. In the afternoon I read the beginning of the 14th chapter of the gospel of John to Steven. "In my Father's house are many rooms. If it were not so, would I have told you that I go to prepare a place for you?"

I explained that Jesus has promised us a home in heaven. I said that we would always be a family. After a minute Steven said, "Can you say that again?" So I explained it again.

In the evening Steven's grandmother, aunt and uncle came for a short visit. At bedtime Steven said, "Can you explain it all to me again?" So I did. And I prayed with him.

On April 23rd Steven was restless. We were in regular communication with our doctor and increased the morphine drip. We received instructions for handling Steven's care.

We tried to find a position of comfort for Steven and asked if he wanted to sit in Dan's lap. He said yes. I encouraged him to rest against his daddy. I asked if he wanted me to hold his hands and he nodded. Then he said, "Mommy, sing."

I sang *Jesus Loves Me* and *Oh, How I Love Jesus*. Steven had a couple more questions about God. Then Steven spoke his last words, "Okay, let's go."

That evening dear friends from our church came to sit with us and pray with us during the final hours of Steven's life. We were with him as he took his last breath.

Our family pulled together to honor Steven's life at the wake and funeral. After the funeral was over Julia said, "It is just like the game isn't it?"

"What do you mean?" I asked.

"It's just like Save the Whales. Steven is in the safe haven, but we are still in the game."

Julia's words lingered in my mind. We had made this journey as a family.

The following days were a challenge. I felt like we were leaving Steven behind, and I struggled with my faith. Over the years I had read books by C.S. Lewis. He wrote about the Christian faith, so I picked up his book, *A Grief Observed*. C.S. Lewis had lost his wife to cancer, and he expressed raw emotion about confronting death. He had doubts. It gave me some comfort to know that C.S. Lewis had also struggled.

I did a word study on the word death and realized that the Bible describes death as painful and ugly. "The last enemy to be destroyed is death." 1 Corinthians 15:26

I read the account of Lazarus' death in the gospel of John, chapter 11. When Jesus arrived in the town of Bethany and saw the grief of Mary and others, he wept. I read the passage again and again. I believe that Jesus was who he said he was, the Son of God. Yet he was acquainted with human grief.

During the summer I read through my journals, and I paused when I read about the days leading up to bone marrow transplant. The words that were given to me in prayer came back to me. *Steven will be okay, but you need to be comforted.*

The nature of God that was shown to me throughout Steven's illness was becoming clearer. As I reviewed my journal I could see the way we were loved. Friends and neighbors became the hands of God. During difficult decisions a pathway opened for us. Steven flourished despite the illness and major medical treatments.

Why didn't God miraculously heal Steven? I don't know, but I do know that God heard my prayers. Steven was loved, and his trust in God grew during illness. Our family was loved.

Over time prayer had become more and more a conversation with God. I learned that it is possible to ask questions. God's desire is for us to communicate with him. I was glad to have my journal because it reminded me of all that God had provided, reasons to give thanks.

A few years later I went back to work as a labor/delivery nurse at a community hospital. There is a similarity between birth and death. It is a fierce physical process. It is a gift of grace to assist in the intimate moments of human transformation—both the birth of new life and the passage into death. God gave me the courage to walk beside my son as he entered eternal life.

All Bible quotes from the English Standard Version, by permission of Crossway Books, Wheaton, IL.

Feeding & Failure
by Christina Chiu

"Vroom! It's an airplane," I say, flying the spoon toward Tyler's mouth.

Tyler laughs, watches it come at his face, and then at the last, most crucial moment, bats it away. Peach puree splats over the floor. While it happens to be lunch time, this ritual actually occurs every morning, noon, and evening since we started transitioning from breast to solids two months ago at 8 months. Peach, pear, broccoli and pear, apple, squash. None of it matters. The answer is always: Not Interested!

It's like this that I get to watch Tyler starve, bit by bit, each day. The doctors "suggestion" to wean seems to be backfiring. Tyler is willing to give up the nursing, but continues to refuse solids. The weigh in at the doctor's office this morning indicates that he's lost another pound the last two weeks. He didn't have an ounce to lose, yet he's lost a pound. He has fallen off the curve; he's now officially termed "failure to thrive."

"Eat," I say, nudging the spoon at his mouth. He presses his lips tight and turns his face away. He flails his arms, knocking the spoon onto the table.

"Tyler!" I feel desperation so great I can no longer contain myself. I love him so much, I want to strangle him. "Fuck!"

Tyler watches, stunned by my reaction, but I can't hold back. I throw the bowl across the room. Puree splatters over the floor and walls. Seven surgeries! I get him through them, nurture him patiently back to health each time. Now *this*.

Strapped in his high chair, Tyler starts crying. I jump up from my seat. From the corner of my eye, I see Tyler stretching his arms toward me. "Ma", "Ma," "Ma."

I race upstairs to my room as Tyler's wails.

My entire body shakes. Rage has taken over. "I didn't sign up for this," I mutter, slamming the door behind me. I grab the pillows from the bed and throw them one by one across the room. "I — never — signed — up — for — *this*!" I pound my fists against the mattress, scream and tear at my hair. The other day, a well intentioned friend tells me, "God only gives what you can handle." Really? I thought. Well, fuck God. Fuck the malicious bastard who did this to my son. It's not fair. Tyler was born VACTERL, an acronym for a rare syndrome of birth defects that stand for vertebral, anal, cardiac, tracheal, esophageal, renal, limbs. He was impacted in all these systems except limbs. The Buddha taught that life is suffering. But why my Tyler?

Why me?

Then I find myself spent and crying. Maybe even praying. Help my baby. Please help him. Whatever it is I did, either in this life or the last, punish me, not him. He's innocent.

Then, suddenly, I stop. It's quiet downstairs. I wipe the tears from my face with my hands, rubbing them on my jeans as I hurry out of the room and back downstairs.

Tyler is seated calmly in his high chair, tears still wet on his face, patting the flat of his palms over the plastic tabletop in front of him. When he sees me, he offers a smile. Peach puree covers his face and hair.

I quickly free him from the seat and take him in my arms. "I'm so sorry," I say, dousing him with kisses. "Mommy's so sorry."

He pats the flat of his peachy palms on my face and in my hair, and chuckles with delight.

My T. He's the light inside all this darkness. As heartbroken and helpless as I feel, he makes me smile. There's hope. In the tantrum of life, he makes me stop, listen, and love again.

Later, I inform the surgeon of the urgency of the feeding situation, and Tyler is scheduled immediately for another swallow study a couple days later. In the meanwhile, there's the daily home health visits, the occupational and physical therapist, a nutritional consult, and a GI visit. The exhaustion's so great, I'm practically dragging myself around, but the Gastroenterologist is very nice and I'm actually looking forward to seeing him. He's funny, and even though I look like shit, he's kind enough to flirt with me. He's what I've termed a "normal." He doesn't wear the stupid white doctor's coat, nor does he don an "I'm so superior" MD identity. More importantly, not only does he make me laugh, but he gives me the chance to make him laugh too.

In his office, the doctor examines Tyler. "Say 'Ah'," he says.

Tyler bangs his trucks together.

"Yeah, I wouldn't either," the doc says. He, too, is concerned about the weight loss. I tell him about the swallow study tomorrow, and he says he'd like to do an endoscopy as well, in order to scope the upper GI tract. Tyler's on Prevacid for reflux, which is common for children who have had esophageal repairs, but if he isn't getting enough medication, the acid may be burning the lining of the esophagus.

Tears gush to my eyes. I should be grateful. It's not surgery. And yet, I worry. He's so little and he's been through so many rounds of anesthesia. The cumulative effect may have negative consequences cognitively.

The doctor sees the tears swelling in my eyes. He sees me trying to hide it from Tyler. He offers me a tissue. I'm sitting beside Tyler on the examination table. "I can't do this," I say, dabbing the tears from my face. "I'm just *so* exhausted."

We watch Tyler play with his trucks on the examination table.

"Are you getting any support?" the doc asks. "Family?"

I think about my parents, whom I'm no longer speaking to because they chose to go on a tour in China when I needed them most, when Tyler was having the tethered spinal cord release. It was his sixth surgery. My husband Cliff couldn't take any more days off from work. We needed someone to stay home with my older son James. Not just someone. Family.

"Support?" I finally reply. "Well, I've got a great nursing bra."

He laughs. It's a moment. A connection.

"I guess you need to nurse to really get it."

"I guess."

When I don't laugh, he adds, "If you'd like to see a psychiatrist, I'd be happy to ask around for you."

"Mm, maybe."

He watches me for a moment. "You've lost some weight."

I consider it for a moment. My clothes do seem roomier than usually. "Maybe, but it doesn't count."

"No, huh?"

"What I've lost in pounds I've gained in inches." Because of Tyler's condition in utero, he didn't swallow the amniotic fluid. It built up. I got so big that my abdominal muscles split apart. For entertainment sake, I push my fingers into the separated area, getting knuckle deep.

"That's impressive," he smiles, listening to Tyler's chest. "A new look."

"Right?" I say. "The preggo look. It's the new 'sexy'."

"Having any sleep issues?" he asks, laughing.

"Maybe, but it doesn't count, either."

"I'm not even going to ask," he says, both hands off.

But he does ask, and when I tell him that I play everything back in my mind all night long, what I did, what I should have done instead, what I need to do now. He suggests medication.

"I hate meds," I say. What I don't tell him is this: Zoloft may be the cause of Tyler's defects. I was on it three weeks before the pregnancy became apparent. I've been researching via internet and there have been class action lawsuits against Pfizer.

"You don't need to take it long term," he says. "Think of it as a temporary respite, just smoothing out the bumps."

"But I'm breastfeeding."

He looks it up in one of his reference books. "No, the amount that gets into the breast milk is minimal," he says. "Out of all of them it's as safe as you're going to get."

"There's just no time. To see someone consistently every week? I mean, it's tough enough getting to all of his appointments."

The doc shifts over to his desk. He scribbles something on a prescription pad, rips off the page, and hands it over.

It's for me: Zoloft, 150 mg per day.

At hospital radiology, I get a lead smock to wear with a thyroid protector. Tyler gets restrained so he can't move. He is literally mummified with duct taped so that his arms are strapped to his sides and his legs immobilized. The nurse turns him onto his side to avoid aspiration. Then she draws the top of the X-ray machine down close to his face. He screams, high pitched, terrified.

"It's okay, sweetheart," I tell him. "I'm here. I'm right here."

The radiologist, surgeon, and nurse vacate the room to protect themselves from radiation. I brought a bottle of breast milk, which the nurse has mixed with barium, and now it's my job to feed it to Tyler. He's getting a procedure called a fluoroscopy, which is a series of X-rays, which, taken together provides a continuous look at the motion and movement of the liquids being swallowed.

The machine powers on. It's loud, and makes the kind of whirring sound I've always equated in my mind with nuclear missile launches. There's a monitor beside me. His skeletal structure appears white, almost ghostly, especially around the edges of the body where the soft tissue is muscle or skin. But the esophagus is clear.

Tyler takes one suck of the barium, then spits it out. A trickle gets swallowed, and I see on the screen a thin black thread, which disperses like smoke down the esophagus. Tyler's screaming so hard that the tremor makes him shake.

"I know," I say, squeezing my face close to his. "I'm sorry." I know inside those restraints he's struggling to bat the bottle away, but can't. He tries to turn his head one way, then the other. The barium drips onto his cheek. He attempts to scream again, and I quickly shove the bottle into his mouth. He continues his vocal tirade, refusing to suck, and then it's me who starts shaking. "It's okay, sweetheart. Just a few sips."

Finally, resigned to the torture, he quiets and drinks the barium solution. Chinese have a term "fang soong," meaning to let go. It's as if I'm seeing his soul give and dissipate. His entire being dims. Suddenly, without his cheery spunk and smile, he seems smaller and so fragile, like a bundle a mother has left at the church doorstep.

I've abandoned him; that's what I've done. As his mother, my duty is to protect and I have failed. I try to squeeze myself closer. "I'm so sorry, sweetheart," I say. "Mommy's so sorry you have to go through this."

Tyler finishes three quarters of the bottle. All-in-all, the procedure takes forty-five minutes. As soon as it's over, the whir of the machine goes silent, the nurse charges back in through the door, and the machine is lifted up and away from Tyler. "Okay, baby," she says, unraveling the duct tape from around his body. His face and hair are drenched with perspiration and his clothes soaked through. "Mommy, do you have a change of clothes for him?" she asks, sanitizing and resetting the area.

I hug Tyler to my body. He reaches for the breast. There's no seating in the room, so I nurse him standing up, my tears dripping onto his face. Tyler nurses are unfazed. Desperately he clings on with his hands. I dry his face.

Through the window, I can see the surgeon and radiologist reviewing the video. Once the surgeon's done, she comes into the room. "That went well," she says.

"Really?" Hope rises in my chest.

"His swallow looks good. I didn't see a stricture."

"So, then," I start. "What next?"

"Let's see what happens with the endoscopy," she says.

I feel myself deflate. Maybe Tyler senses it, too, because he unlatches from my breast. I take the opportunity to change him, unfolding the changing mat on the counter. An endoscopy would mean another overnight prep, hours in the morning when the baby will be screaming to be nursed while Mommy stands there saying "No." It'll mean anesthesia, another morning facing a black hole as he gets wheeled into the OR without me. I lay him on the changing mat.

"Full diaper," the surgeon notices.

"It's from all the screaming," I say. "It's like there's pressure in his system."

The surgeon nods as if to say, "Interesting." She tells me to make an appointment in the White Plains office once we get results for the endoscopy, then leaves for another appointment upstairs.

After changing his diaper, I dig out a spare set of clothes. "Little Brother," the T-shirt says.

The radiological assistant arrives. "Would you mind doing that outside?" she asks.

My temperature spikes. I stop what I'm doing and turn my full attention on her. "Yes, I would mind," I say, in a low, steady voice. "I would mind very much."

"I'm sorry, but we need the room for the next patient."

I've been told that I have a gaze that can intimidate. Maybe it's true because she backs off, saying, "I'll be back," and leaves the room.

Swallow study. Endoscopy. Ruling out possibilities this way proves futile. The surgeon discusses putting the G-tube back again. Tenths. Quarter ounces. Every ounce Tyler loses, my soul dies a little more. Eat! God damn it, eat! Every time I raise my voice to this little being, I hate myself all the more. I revisit the idea of God. What is God?

If God exists, where is it?

I give in and start Zoloft, plodding forward one day at a time. But the fatigue. It's in-my-bones familiar. So familiar, it's terrifying. Two years ago, I 'm diagnosed with Amyloidosis, a rare disease that occurs when one's bone marrow produces abnormal protein that cannot be broken down by the body, and so, gets lodged in an organ instead. Over time, the buildup of amyloid can cause organ failure. The local hematologist recommends immediate chemo and bone marrow transplant, the standard course of treatment, but since I have been living with this condition for more than 15 years, during which my life grows gradually more myopic, I can't help but question not only the diagnosis but what the rush is. James is six and in Kindergarten. Do I really want to destroy my bone marrow?

The top Amyloid expert is at the Mayo Clinic. I get a second opinion there. The doctor confirms the diagnosis. I ask if I can try alternative methods first. He agrees on the condition that I return in six months, and if the bone marrow is still producing abnormal protein, that I proceed with the treatment. As soon as I get home, I research and start a tapping protocol, Reiki, colonics, and also change my diet. Within months, I feel so good, so energetic, and probably better than I have ever felt in my life. Miraculously, when I return to Mayo, the tests indicate that the bone marrow is no longer producing abnormal protein. "Whatever you're doing, keep doing it," he says. "See you in two years."

I never go back, though, because I get pregnant. Then, I postpone because of Tyler's condition and the surgeries. Now, maybe it's too late.

The next morning, the home health aid arrives to help with the colostomy change. We go through the motions, removing the bag, cleaning the area, drying it, reapplying a new barrier, and finally, the colostomy bag itself. We have come to know a little about one another. She lost her house in the financial crises, and yet, here she is helping me with Tyler in my six-bedroom Tudor in Scarsdale. Today, I must look especially bad because she says, "Why don't you go lie down for a while," she says.

I look at the clock. She's only supposed to be here for an hour and we've spent the first 45 minutes administering to Tyler. "You're leaving soon," I say.

"It's fine," she says. "My patient this afternoon had to cancel. She has a doctor's appointment. So I'm in no rush today."

Normally, I'd find such grace and kindness incredibly moving. Today, I feel strangely numb. "Thank you," I say.

In my room, I lie back in bed, close my eyes, and the world vanishes.

I wake up foggy. Then I realize two hours have passed and hurry to Tyler's room. Tyler's sitting on her lap as she rocks back and forth in the nursing chair. "Why didn't you wake me?" I say, mortified.

"It's fine," she says.

"No, it's not."

"Consider it a gift."

"Thanks." I smile, feeling a flicker of gratitude. A little sleep can go a long way.

"Feel better?" she asks.

"Yes," I say. However, my body still feels like a ten-ton brick. "Sort of."

I take the baby from her. After she leaves, I finally call the Mayo Clinic. The medical coordinator tells me it will take a few days to arrange with the doctor, it will require procedures and tests in other departments, but she will contact me as soon as she finds a date and makes the necessary arrangements.

A month later, I'm at Mayo. It's a three day interlude. The Monday afternoon is travel, check-in, and getting reacquainted with the hospital and its many buildings. According to the itinerary, Tuesday and Wednesdays are packed with appointments, literally arranged back to back, so there's no time for things like getting lost. It's what I requested. I fly home Wednesday evening because Tyler has doctor's appointments Thursday and Friday. Thanks to Early Intervention, he also has physical therapy, he started rolling late because of the colostomy, which delayed his walking, and most importantly, he has a new feeding therapist. I can't allow a delay.

Monday night in the hotel, I get to sleep early. Despite pumping every four hours, I wake the next morning feeling rested.

My office visit with the doctor isn't until Wednesday morning. He wants labs, first. Cardiology, pulmonary, hematology, and endocrinology. Gastroenterology will do a colonoscopy after I see him. I'm familiar with the tests, not only from my own experience, but from Tyler's. Tuesday afternoon, they put me under general anesthesia in order to get a bone marrow biopsy. What this entails is jamming a needle through the back of the hip bone. I've actually experienced this particular biopsy awake; the experience was so traumatic that I'm grateful and relieved I don't have to bear witness to it again.

After all the appointments, I'm exhausted by the time I return to the hotel. Because of the colonoscopy tomorrow, I've had nothing to eat. All day, I've been drinking apple juice and water. Now, it's time for the laxative. I gulp it down, and despite the numerous visits to the bathroom all night, along with pumping every four hours, I sleep so well that I wake up feeling the best I've felt in a long time. I walk into the doctor's office already knowing that I'm okay. "There's no evidence of recurrent localized amyloidosis," he states.

"I know," I smile. "Do I still need the colonoscopy?"
"I recommend you get it," he says.

"What if they see a something?"

"Let's proceed accordingly."

I hurry to Gastroenterology. They gown me. Before they start an IV for anesthesia, a resident reminds me of all the DOs and DON'T DOs following the procedure. "Refrain from driving or operating heavy machinery," she says.

"It's lucky I'm flying and not driving," I say.

"Oh, no," she says. "No flying."

"You're joking."

She stares straight at me.

"But I have to get home tonight," I say, briefly explaining about Tyler and his condition.

"If you have an adverse reaction from the anesthesia during a flight, it would not be possible to get immediate medical attention."

"Can I get the colonoscopy without anesthesia?" I ask. "Do people ever do that?"

"Oh," she says. "Yes, that's doable. It happens on occasion."

"It's not super painful is it?"

"If it becomes unbearable, we can administer anesthesia then," she says.

We proceed with the colonoscopy. I lie on my side and watch the monitor mounted on the wall. The doctor moves the scope rapidly through the colon. The tissue is pink and slick with moisture. It's a tunnel, ribbed with muscle. I feel the pressure of the probe in my gut, but it doesn't hurt—at least not until it arrives at the transverse colon where there's a sharp curve. The probe knocks against the tissue. My abdomen automatically cramps up.

"Oh," I groan.

But the scope moves swiftly and the pain passes. Two years ago, the GI who discovered the "mass", which turned out to be the amyloid, described it as being "embedded within three inches of the colon." So far, the tissue is pink and healthy. I wait for the amyloid, which we never removed.

The scope arrives at the next bend. The pain makes my entire body tense. The cramping feels like the earlier stages of labor. Then it rounds the corner and continues onward.

"That's it," the doctor announces.

"But where's the amyloid?" I ask. "There was an amyloid."

The doctor shrugs. On the monitor are screenshots of different segments of my colon.

It's gone. I healed myself.

That night, I'm at home nursing Tyler in the rocking chair. Cliff told me Tyler refused to eat or take the bottle while I was gone, opting to drink water instead. I said the new feeding therapist starts tomorrow, so there's hope, yet I can tell just from holding Tyler that he's lost more weight, which would usually terrify me, except that the time away, while not exactly a vacation, proved to be a much needed break.

Tyler glances up from the breast at me, and giggles.

"What's so funny?" I laugh, which opens a trapdoor to my heart and nearly makes me cry. I feel so moved by the ebb and flow of joy and love, and sadness. Why T?

Why me?

Because I can help him, I realize. Life is suffering. I realize I have held a wrong view about what the Buddha was trying to say. What he was saying was that with one, there is always the other. With suffering there is happiness; with happiness there is suffering. Everything is impermanent and always changing, and it's our attachment to either of these that begets more suffering.

Suddenly, it all makes karmic sense. *I healed myself before; I can heal Tyler now.* I think about all the events that led to this moment. For me to heal Tyler, I need to believe I can heal. And in fact, as the colonoscopy proved, I had healed. In order to have the confidence to believe that I have that power, I needed to be awake to see the colonoscopy. The only reason I refused anesthesia was because of the flight. But to get to this Mayo in the first place, I needed to feel exhausted and sick.

So then was feeling exhausted and sick such a "bad" thing after all? If I leap back farther, is getting sick with the Amyloidosis a "bad" thing if the methods I learn can ultimately help my son now? In the end, these experiences provided the path to possible solutions. Only now do I see that from darkness and despair there can grow hope and healing.

That is God. The way of the Buddha.

We Are On The Floor Talking
by Jean Colgan Gould

1.

"You know that crazy wallpaper?" he is saying.

"Wallpaper?" I say, retrieving a blanket from the bed.

"You know." He grins with all those perfect teeth, with his rosy cheeks, stretching out the word 'know.'

I am lying next to him now on the carpet in our bedroom.

"You remember," he insists, raising his voice just a bit. "The guy refused to hang the wallpaper."

My head rests on the edge of his pillow. I lick his ear lobe. "Let's do it one more time," I say.

"I love that wallpaper," he says. "The guy told you it was too busy for the room. You made him hang it anyway. You were wonderful."

We are on the floor talking, waiting, whispering. Irving has fallen again. The hospice nurse is on the way, but it is the middle of the night in a January freeze. A foot of new snow has been plowed and shoveled, but the roads remain icy.

"Maybe we should call 911," I say. I sit up. "They'd be here in a few minutes."

He looks up at the closet we share. "Give everything to the poor," he says.

Even if you say you only need help lifting your husband off the floor, the 911 people will send a fire engine and Emergency Medical Teams, creating a whirlwind when they mean to project safety. We will wait.

"Are you warm enough?" I say. We hold hands. It is hard to tell whose fingers are whose.

Of course, he is warm enough. We have the thermostat in the room at eighty degrees. I have lately called it the desert. Still, he wears a sweater over his flannel pajamas.

He is dying. But he is not dying this minute. He has only forgotten he is too weak to navigate on his own and has dropped to the floor. It is impossible to call this an emergency. Besides, just now he is comfortable. We will not call 911. We will lie here and talk and hold each other until the nurse gets here. If the sun rises before then, I will phone a neighbor. And tomorrow I will order a hospital bed and raise the sides at night.

"Where did you find that wallpaper anyway?" he is saying.

I had not wanted to confine him during his last days. But even under pain-relieving medications, he is restless. He is characteristically restless. Why did I imagine that a man whose mantra is 'Let's go. Let's go. The green light's on.' would remain still?

But just now, he is going nowhere. We are lying on the floor.

"My legs still work," he is saying, raising one then the other off the floor, "except for standing and walking."

"That's true," I say."

He had been on his way to the tiny bathroom, only steps from the bed, where the wallpaper under discussion shouts its pink, purple, green marks on a white background. Like children's finger-painting, I always thought. Perhaps in the context of Irving's condition, it exists as a small triumph.

"Yes," he whispers, "let's do it," he says, "one more time."

We giggle, though the sounds are brief and murmured.

2.

"You have great muscle tone," he said, the first time he took me in his arms.

Introduced by mutual friends, we'd met playing tennis. He had never known a woman like me, he said, a woman who would run every ball down, a woman with such terrific ground strokes. I should be playing tournaments, he said. And, he said, he'd been divorced for six months and hadn't met anyone yet.

He is fourteen years older than I am. He is Jewish. I am Catholic. He's a businessman, a capitalist. I'm an academic, a poet. But we both wear clothing from L.L. Bean. Our politics are similarly left of center. And, of course, there's the tennis.

Two years later, we marry. For a time, our four teenage children live with us. Though I make a chart with cooking and household assignments, this is not successful. We survive anyway. In fact, I do start playing local tennis tournaments. Not only that, I begin publishing my writing. Irving buys me an electric typewriter. My first novel is published.

"You can do anything," my husband tells me. He calls me Your Highness.

Now we lie on the floor, waiting, alone in the pre-dawn hours on a wintry night. I have promised he will never have to go to a nursing home.

But it can take a long time to die. A lifetime.

A decade before, when Irving is diagnosed with prostate cancer, he is so cavalier about it that I go off to the Himalayas while he has forty-two radiation treatments. His point of reference for discomfort and danger, after all, is the South Pacific during the Second World War. He keeps working, drives himself to the Massachusetts General Hospital every day of expertly focused radiation and recovers. He served for three years with the United States Marines in the Philippines. "A little cancer is nothing," he says.

By the time I come home, two months later, his hair has already begun to grow back. He meets me at the airport as usual. Though he rarely speaks of the war, I know that he was so happy to get out of it in one piece that he never wants to leave home again.

So while I am seeking out places off the map, he installs a wood stove or new windows in the house, spends time with his large extensive family, and, of course, continues working. My mother is the only one with guts enough to ask if there is something wrong with our marriage, but I suppose others also wonder at our lack of what they would call togetherness.

"I do all the exploring I want via the National Geographic," Irving often says.

I am still teaching and writing. My second book is published. And a third one.

Irving is diagnosed with a late-stage lymphoma. After several rounds of a complicated chemotherapy regimen, he recovers. But I stay home for this one. Despite its renowned expertise and support, the Dana Farber Cancer Institute is in a sobering place. The ordeal is rigorous.

We check in for each appointment among patients with masks, in wheelchairs; patients who have lost their hair, are emaciated. Every staff member has eye contact. Patients do not.

The chemicals are administered by special nurses wearing thick purple rubber gloves. Irving lies back in a lounge chair while the IV is plugged into his arm. He talks about the Red Sox or looks at the sports page while I work on the Times puzzle. Each treatment takes a long time, several hours.

The side effects are terrible. I once thought that the purple gloves were to protect patients from possible contamination, but I realize the nurses do not want to come in contact with the dangerous chemicals dripping into my husband's body.

At home, we smoke marijuana to combat the nausea. It doesn't help. I bake custard in individual cups Irving eats with a wooden spoon. Even the metal in his teeth feels corrosive. His red blood cell count plummets after every treatment. There is an antidote that renders him exhausted though alive. He loses his hair and thirty pounds. At the bank for a transaction, his trousers actually fall down. We use a necktie for a belt. Yet, however thin and often tired, with an office in the house, he works. He recovers and will live seven more years.

We invent a new short-court tennis game. He designs a website for his business. I dig out my passport.

3.

The hospice folks suggest a chaplain. This is not a good idea.

My husband and I have both been disappointed by the religious institutions of our early days. Even before we met, the rules created by men in high places turned us away, made us irreverent. Yet vestiges of our upbringing remain. If Irving is a secular Jew, I suppose I am a secular Catholic. Separately and together, we have railed against orthodoxy of any kind.

And then--believe it or not--here we are one clear spring morning on the campus of Brandeis University, approaching the Bethlehem Chapel. As we make our way to the small building across the grass, Irving leans on the cane he uses now.

It is five years after his recovery from lymphoma. He has recently had a knee replacement--and a heart attack.

"This must be your husband," a woman says at the door. "Welcome."

I do not remember her name. She and several others guide us to comfortable seats in the chapel where about seventy or eighty people are talking quietly. Close to the altar, a young man plays a guitar.

The congregation stands for the opening hymn. The priest walks down the aisle. And the mass begins. Actually, before the Sign of the Cross starting the liturgy, the priest turns to the assembled group.

"Welcome to all," he says. He is a man in his sixties, on this Sunday in green vestments. "Welcome to all Catholics and non-Catholics, those who are divorced, gay or straight, those of other faith traditions: our Jewish and Muslim sisters and brothers. Whether you are a believer of orthodoxy or are just hanging on by your fingernails, we are glad to have you with us this morning."

It is the fingernail comment that most draws me to this group. We might all be fingernailers. It doesn't matter.

Irving and I hold hands. The liturgy proceeds with its readings and prayers and music. Irving stands and sits and sings softly. He had wanted "to see what it was all about." His face gives no clue to his thoughts, and when it is time for communion, he rises and follows me in the line down the aisle. He takes the wafer, puts it in his mouth and chews it up.

Of course, in pre-Vatican II days, this would be a serious offense, a mortal sin. And now? I don't know or care. Irving wanted to come here with me. I hope the experience satisfies his curiosity and provides some comfort.

In the car, on the way home, he says, "It's all about love, isn't it?"

After the service, he and the priest, Father Walter Cuenin, chatted as they sipped coffee on the pebbled path by the chapel doors. Irving talked about the founding of Brandeis just after the war, how it had grown. Walter spoke of the invitation the school offered him to become its Catholic chaplain after he had been ousted from his large suburban parish by the Boston Archdiocese hierarchy.

Of course, I think to myself, it makes perfect sense that I would connect with a Catholic community on the campus of a Jewish university led by a renegade priest.

Irving rattles on about the details of Brandeis' origins and development, interspersed with remarks about what a fine man Walter is, how glad he is that he has come with me.

Walter Cuenin was among those priests who signed a letter to Cardinal Bernard Law to stop protecting sexually abusive priests. Of course, he had also spoken out for the rights of all people, including women. The archdiocese had to silence him.

I had been making the rounds of Boston-area Catholic churches for several years after a particularly disturbing trip to rural Bolivia when the two of us met. I had traveled with a Quaker group to visit and to assess the efficacy of projects it funded.

Having witnessed a horrifying number of questionable actions by missionaries of varying Christian faiths that seemed designed to keep the indigenous population in "its place," I found it necessary to take a look at ethical issues among organized religions. Strangely enough, the only seminaries in Boston offering courses on morality and ethics were Catholic. So after a very long absence from the Church, I began my investigation with the Jesuits.

As Irving and I wind our way down the hill and out of the gates of the university, I see that the magnolias are just past their early bloom. Petals drift to the softening earth. A few whirl in a gentle breeze.

"Nature teaches us everything," I say.

Irving nods. It is not a new insight. These recent years, I have learned that religious institutions are evolving--or they are dying--sometimes both. Zealots shout and threaten. Some give women bibles instead of birth control information. But goodness endures. Perhaps it endures side-by-side with suffering. But it endures. A magnolia blossom can teach us this, if we are open to it.

Any cultural/religious differences between my husband and me, I see now, were superseded by the length and depth of our bond. I was raised to consider the "preferential option for the poor" above all else, while Irving's tradition put family first.

Neither of these priorities is so terrible except perhaps in the extreme. I'm a bleeding heart. And Irving would be the first to acknowledge his family has a command performance every five minutes. Are these Catholic or Jewish traits? In the face of life-threatening illness, they no longer matter.

And though it was the perversions of doctrine that turned me upside down in Latin America, these were exactly what sent me back into the arms of my religious origins. And though my husband will not attend Mass with me again, I am grateful I can share its positive aspects with him during his final years.

4.

We are on the floor, waiting.

I had promised my husband there would be no pain or nursing home or anxiety. And just now there is only the waiting.

In the end, though we had lately been told he had congestive heart failure and a variety of other complications, it is the prostate cancer that is killing Irving. When you sign up for radiation treatments, you don't know--and no one bothers to tell you--that ten years later, you will likely suffer from radiation cystitis, that the lining of the bladder will fall away, be unable to pass through the uterus, resulting in excruciating pain.

Such is the pain that causes us to move hospice into place. Still, it takes twenty-four hours before the state approves the morphine prescription. Fortunately I have been stock-piling medications for years in anticipation of just such a time. But only the anti-anxiety pills appear to calm Irving. I feel like downing a handful of them myself.

He was sitting at the breakfast table eating his usual oatmeal and blueberries with cream when he rose and excused himself. Was he using a walker? Possibly

I remained there drinking black coffee and reading the paper. All our excitement was directed toward the election of Barak Obama who would be sworn in as President in a matter of days.

The sound from the other end of the house was neither a scream nor a cry. It was like nothing I had ever heard. I was beside my husband before it ended.

"Give me the pill!" Irving shouted when I found him doubled over.

We had joked in the gallows-humor way people do when death seems inevitable about there being a single pill that would do the deed when the time came. Of course, such pills were only the fantasies of spy novels.

Irving's face had lost its color. Even his blue eyes appeared faded.

I helped him to the bed.

When I got the doctor on the phone, having claimed an emergency, she agreed it was time to call hospice. Three weeks before, when Irving had been released from the Brigham and Women's Hospital, we had settled on just such a contingency plan, even though one physician at the hospital had said Irving "looks great and will probably last another year."

In my experience, doctors are reluctant to speak of death as if such an outcome is a failure on their part. Even Irving did not want to go anywhere near the word itself. And maybe I'm just looking for trouble to insist on naming the events so affecting us. But there are worse things than death.

At first when I uttered this statement, I guess I expected a response, but when Irving--and later, others--said nothing, I generally continued. "Worse things." Pause. "Like pain. Like anxiety." And then I let it go, hoping the seeds I was planting might take root.

Not that I wanted him or anyone else to die before their time. But I'm against suffering. We could defuse the fear, in my opinion, by naming it. As I said, I let it go.

"I forgot to bang the pan," he said.

Instead of a bell, I had placed a spoon and frying pan on the night table for him to alert me. I knew he'd never use it. I also knew his pain had not diminished.

"What would I do without you?" he said.

The nurse assigned to us for post-hospital care arrived within a half-hour for a previously scheduled visit and absorbed the panic I could only admit in the next minutes as we waited for the hospice people.

"On a scale of ten," she said, posing the usual question, "what's your level of pain?"

"Are you kidding?" Irving shouted. He flung his arms away from his body. "This is worse than the war!"

Time has a way of stretching and shrinking and scrambling during a crisis. It can envelope you, become liquid, harden, or simply stop before slipping away.

Home health care requires a precarious balance of need and treatment. The schedule of nurses, health aides, physical and occupational therapists, as well as and occasional social worker can feel invasive. For several weeks now, each had documented her visit in a folder kept on our dining table.

With the advent of the hospice team, the traffic would double.

5.

When Irving decided to have a knee replacement several years before this, we were confident about the outcome. He was eighty then, but had made a great recovery from both prostate cancer and lymphoma. He'd had a hip replacement some years before this with no difficulties. And though he had lately given up driving, this had not slowed him in any way. He hired a driver and continued working. We were not worried about the surgery.

Yet a day or two afterward, the "little indigestion" he mentioned turned out to be a serious heart attack. He was placed in intensive care for several weeks and subsequently transferred to a rehabilitation center. In addition, he had not fully recovered from the anesthesia administered during the knee replacement. He was disoriented and often confused. Such reactions are common among older patients, I was told. It would pass.

For several months he remained at the rehab center without significant progress. Some days when I visited, I would find him in a group of patients coloring butterflies on a mimeographed sheet of paper with a crayon. Nevertheless, he remained in good spirits, except to say that the orderlies did not respond when he rang to be escorted to the bathroom.

One wintry day, not unlike this current one, against medical orders, I decided it was time to bring him home.

"You can't do that," they told me. "He can't walk. He needs twenty-four hour care."

That morning, having bought enough groceries for a month, I wheeled my husband out of rehab into my car. We drove home through a storm. To avoid stairs, I dragged the wheelchair through the snow to the back of the house. Pulling it over the threshold of a sliding glass door, I got Irving inside. The adrenalin of a successful escape coursed through my body. I lifted my husband into an arm chair and pointed my finger at him.

"Don't you dare move," I said.

For several days, he followed my instructions. I was able to help him up and down, into and out of bed. But inevitably he fell and firefighters righted him after I called 911.

Thus began our intermittent connection with the Visiting Nurse Association. Irving recovered. He began working again. His knee healed. His mind cleared. But he would deny heart problems. He refused cardiac medications as well as the stringent dietary restrictions. He would live his life "as a person, not an invalid."

Sometime during this period, he quietly gave away his tennis things, making no mention of it to me, and never once complaining when I went off to play.

He read more. Always a history and political junkie, he shouted at the TV news. We both followed the Celtics. Still, much of the time he spent in his office working on the new website or arranging sales calls.

Having been diagnosed with macular degeneration, at some point during these months, I began having treatment at the Massachusetts Eye and Ear Infirmary. And though another time this may have been a daunting enterprise, I drove myself into and out of the city, frequently getting injections in both eyes. Always concerned about what I'd find at home, I held my breath until I got there, but more often than not, Irving would have dinner in the oven and a glass of wine in hand for me.

Nevertheless, my own heart pounded each time I turned the corner onto our street. I was more vulnerable after the eye injections, of course. But whether I was returning from teaching or tennis or some other activity, I was uneasy. Often, Irving would be out on a business call with his driver, a man about half Irving's size in his twenty-year old Oldsmobile. Close to the same age, the men had gotten to be fast friends.

When *Forty Years Since my Last Confession*, my memoir about returning to the Catholic Church, was published, Irving's family said it was my best book so far. He bought a hundred copies and gave them out to customers and business associates like candy.

6.

It was a strange time in the Church. The sex abuse tragedy had become public. People inside and outside of the Church took sides. The Boston hierarchy hid behind its authority. Clearly it was no time to feel comfortable being Catholic.

In the 1980s I read a book by Peter Occhiogrosso called *Once a Catholic* that had me nodding in agreement on most pages. Well-known and not-so-well-known current and former Catholics spoke about the influence of the Church on their lives. The upshot was that once a Catholic, always a Catholic. That such a book proved insightful only underscored the extent of my alienation from the Church at that time.

It was probably no accident then that I began my first novel with the protagonist in a confessional. The imagery came easily and powerfully even though I had no notion of myself either as Catholic or particularly spiritual.

But within a few years, as a result of my Himalayan journeys, I would find myself involved with all-things Buddhist. The stillness of meditation, the silence held me as I made my way through mountains and small villages. Himalayans abided with nature, while westerners so often tried to conquer it. The chants and rituals were full of respect and awe.

Much later, when I returned to the Church, I would miss that kind of silence. In efforts to be more communal, more relevant, I suspect, the powers that be had altered the Catholic mass. It was noisier, more interactive.

I was drawn to ritual: offering as it does a respite from the world, though ultimately it has been the rituals of nature that have fed me: the seasons and their certainties of beauty and rebirth.

We lie on the carpet, waiting. Icicles clatter like bones by the windows as the wind knocks at them. There are no soothing rituals to survive nights like this one.

"When I was a boy," Irving is saying.

"You're still a boy," I kiss his cheek.

"When I was a boy," he repeats, "I used to dream of a little blonde girl running down the hill on our street."

I know the story.

"She had curly hair with a ribbon in it," he says. "She was you."

It did no good to point out that my hair is straight.

"I was always waiting for you." This is what he says.

It's enough to break your heart or fill it so much it will burst.

Mercifully, the doorbell rings.

"Don't go anywhere, I say.

My legs are stiff as I rise.

A blast of cold air smacks against my face before I open my mouth to greet the hospice nurse, the night nurse, the emergency nurse.

She is a small woman wrapped in a khaki coat several sizes too large. Stepping inside, she removes her boots and surveys the rooms before dropping her coat on the floor. So far she has said nothing.

"This is our first day of hospice," I say. "Thank you for coming."

I see that she is not just small, barely five feet tall, but also--what's the word?--puffy, as if she might herself be on medication. Cortisone maybe.

Is this a person who will be able to help me lift my husband?

"Where is he?" she says, her features somehow gathering in the center of her face.

"Follow me, "I say, leading her down the hallway.

"The driving is terrible," she says.

This is her job. I do not say this. This is her job: to come out in the middle of the night to assist the dying. "I hope they are paying you double time," I say.

"Are you a Celtics fan?" Irving chirps from the floor as we enter the bedroom.

The woman does not respond.

"OK," I say. "We just need to lift him to the bed."

The nurse places one hand on her hip and the other on her back. I can see this will not be as easy as I expected.

"You take one arm," I say, squatting and getting myself in position.

She bends over. I can see at once that If this woman squats, she will never get up without assistance.

Irving rolls his eyes. The corners of his mouth turn up. "I'll help you," he says, Irving who is too weak now to lift an arm, much less a leg. How can he look so good and be so sick?

The nurse looks at Irving. She eyes the bed. She sighs. "We need to call 911," she says in defeat.

The firefighters arrive in less than five minutes in their rubber coats, boots and brimmed hats. They arrive amid their ubiquitous smiles and good cheer. And I think the house may burst with it. Dwarfing the nurse, without missing a beat, they raise Irving from the floor and place him in bed.

"Is that OK?" one says softly.

Another man adjusts the pillows, smoothes out the blankets. "How you doing, sir?"

"You guys Celtics fans?" says the patient.

"You bet," says the first guy.

And then, they are gone.

The nurse checks my husband's vital signs, but he is sleeping now. She records the information in the hospice notebook. And then, she, too, leaves, driving off into the still-dark night, her tires beating their rhythm against the icy pathways.

I am angry. I didn't want her to stay, but I am irritated by her leaving. There is no rule, of course, that says you have to like the hospice caregivers. And this one probably did not expect a call in the middle of the night.

But we waited hours for her. And then we needed the fire department anyway. Should I have known better? What had I expected? There are no dress rehearsals for this circumstance.

Across the street, light glimmers against the last of this long night. I breathe in and out, hoping those creatures outdoors are managing the cold. The image of a swan, its head tucked under its ample wing, comes to me as a dream. You can pound your fists against the night, and still, the sun rises.

7.

Swiftly and with a astonishing precision, the hospital bed is delivered and assembled shortly after nine that morning.

The hospice nurse arrives and apologizes for her stand-in before adjusting the bed sheets, checking vital signs and taking the time to chat with me at length, offering the compassion I must have been hoping for the previous night.

A home health aide arrives. A Ugandan, he is tall and handsome and well-spoken. He calls Irving "Papa."

Somehow, more snow is falling. A neighbor shovels our walk. Another works on the driveway.

The phone rings and rings.

I am sitting next to my husband in what is now clearly "the sickroom." Medical materials abound. Basins. Sponges. Special disinfectants. The frying pan and its spoon are gone.

If the previous night dragged on and on, during these moments time stands still as deer in headlights.

"Do I have a pulse?" Irving says. "Am I still alive?"

"That's not funny," I say.

The home health aide's name is Victor. A Ugandan named Victor? Maybe not.

"See. Victor thinks it's funny," says Irving.

So his name is Victor.

"You know," Irving is saying, "she saved my life." And he tells a favorite and mostly concocted tale about how I rescued him from the clutches of women who were up to no good.

"Yes, Papa," says Victor.

My feet are cold. I regard them in their wool socks and sheepskin slippers. Such a gentleman, my husband polished his shoes every morning before leaving the house. He placed a clean linen handkerchief in his pocket.

"Give everything to the poor." He said this only the previous night.

And then, as the hospice bluster for the morning ebbs, only the TV voices are before us. But the inauguration of the first African-American President is no longer the most important event in the world.

I am thumbing through the newspaper for the crossword. Irving sleeps. The nurse beckons from the doorway.

At the dining table, a small box of medicines has been placed alongside the continuing care notebooks. Other medicines--one in case of choking, I am told--are in the refrigerator. The morphine is administered by dropper into the mouth and is directly absorbed by the tissues.

"He does not need to swallow the morphine," she says, waiting until I look at the small vial.

"I see," I say.

"Do not be afraid," the nurse says. "It is not the morphine that will kill Irving. It is the disease."

I try swallowing in order to take this in. Eleanor--I will never forget her name--has blond lashes and green eyes. She sets a cup of coffee before me. I wonder if the morphine has a flavor. And then she is gone.

A man in Baghdad sells nightingales from a small shop, cleaning their cages each morning. before hanging them outdoors for customers. I read this in the morning paper. I wonder what a nightingale looks like and go online to find out.

Maybe most days begin with such routines: getting birds ready for sale, or reading the newspaper.

The real story today is that the nightingale man is taken, swept off by enemies he doesn't know, burned, bruised or broken by a troop of angry men who set fire to his shop. And oh, what of those fine but ordinary-looking birds singing in their cages?

Once when I was in an art gallery in Pakistan, a small brown bird flew in through a window. The creature flailed about, looking for escape, while the proprietor assured me that it is good luck to have a bird enter your house.

I am sitting by my husband's side again.

He wakes. "I had the most wonderful dream," he says. "I was running. Imagine. If I could run again." He sleeps.

Lately, I feel as if an animal--a bird--is trapped inside me, knocking against my ribs, desperate to escape. I have never had a running dream. But sometimes, I fly. Sometimes, I soar and soar and soar, or so it seems. Dreams only last a few minutes, they say.

8.

We lie on the floor waiting, holding one another, talking, whispering.

"Who will take care of me?" I say.

"Ha!" he says. "You're a young chick. You'll find someone right away."

Right," I say. "Match-dot-com."

For some weeks now, when I feel myself sagging, I sing hymns. "Onward Christian Soldiers." "A mighty Fortress is Our God." Occasionally, a college fight song demands expression. But mostly I allow myself the comfort of spirituals. "Swing Low, Sweet Chariot."

I am nothing like a young chick. In two weeks I will be seventy years old. I do not want "to find someone right away."

Of course, the question was unfair.

Who will take care of me?

I will take care of myself, as always. Just as Irving has taken care of himself.

Give everything to the poor.

It is the sharing, not interdependence that defined our connection. We have never lived in each other's pockets.

You're a young chick.

Even now, our bond cut both ways: sadness tinged with wit. Humor just a step from tears.

Clearly it is possible to feel more than one thing at a time. Buddhists speak of "being in the moment." But this, I think, precludes neither past nor visions for the future.

Irving will die. The hospice people, the visiting nurse crew will clear out. The hospital bed will be removed. I will indeed give everything in my husband's closet to the poor. I will close down his business, clean out his office. Eventually, I will even get out my passport and take off for Africa.

Someone once asked Irving if I were his daughter. We joked about it, but he never let it go.

The flavor of some moments can last a long time.

During his last hospitalization, when a nurse asked me who I was, I assumed that it related to the age difference. But it turned out to be something else.

"You're the wife?" she said. "The wife? But you're so nice to each other," she said. "So polite."

Later, I reflected that crises provide opportunities. Certainly Irving and I had had our share of quarrels and fits of temper. Neither of us was an easy person. No one who knew us well would use the word 'nice' to describe him or me. But for the most part, we had--individually and together--risen to the occasion of his health challenges.

And that winter night on the floor in our bedroom, we are giddy with relief. We have made it to the final stretch of this long battle. And just now, the prize belongs to us.

My Father's Stroke
by Nancy Gerber

When I heard my father had suffered a stroke, I didn't really understand what that meant. If I thought about the word "stroke," what came to mind were expressions such as " a stroke of genius," or "a stroke of luck," or " with the stroke of a pen." I had no understanding of stroke as a catastrophic illness. I had no idea that stroke stops blood flow to the brain, causes paralysis, destroys short-term memory.

The other day at the town health department, I saw a flyer that said stroke is the number-three leading killer of Americans and I flinched as I remembered how little I knew about stroke in the fall of 1995. What I know now could fill a book.

The losses from my father's stroke plagued him for nearly six years. By the time of his death, on June 17, 2001, he had lost his ability to walk, his kidney function, his short-term memory, most of his eyesight, and his entire left leg. During the last few days of his life, while in the throes of a fatal staphylococcus infection, he finally lost his will to live. I think the rest of us had given up long before he did.

My father was seventy-three when he had the stroke and was self-employed as a CPA, a certified public accountant. He did not have long-term care insurance. He had not made provisions for the sale or transfer of his accounting practice. He was imagining retirement but had planned to keep working part-time for a few more years. He was hoping to travel with my mother.

The day before he had the stroke, he was a gregarious, vital man—father, grandfather, husband, paterfamilias, breadwinner, tennis player, bridge partner, and friend. The day after the stroke, he was someone else. It happened that fast. It was obvious he would never work again, yet it's odd how the mind works: I both knew and didn't know this was the case. As with any devastating accident, it takes a very long time for the mind to grasp what the heart already knows: from now on, everything will be radically different.

I found it difficult to accept my father's disability, the wheelchair and his sudden physical dependence. Even worse was the erosion of his personality. During the months and years that followed the stroke, he became unrecognizable to those who knew and loved him.

Physically, he was altered indeed; he had aged decades in one night. His fringe of gray hair went white, his left arm and leg withered from paralysis, his face slackened, and the rest of his body grew round and soft from paralysis.

His humor disappeared. In place of the sociable, active man I knew was a withdrawn, silent, hostile double.

There is no language to describe such a loss. We have no prayers or rituals for the death of someone who hasn't died.

My father's stroke occurred in the office of one of his clients. At 2:30 on September 18, 1995, my father crumpled in a heap and slid off his chair onto the floor.

The office staff panicked; they thought he had had a heart attack. Someone phoned Emergency Medical Services, who arrived and wanted to take my father to the nearest emergency room. The EMS people could tell he had had a stroke. His blood pressure was very high, his mouth sagged, his speech was slurred. My father refused to go to the ER and joked about his condition. The EMS people hesitated. They knew this was no joke but they were not required to force my father against his will. So they left.

The office staff was very worried. They called my mother, who was at home in New Jersey. She phoned my brother, who worked a few blocks away from my father. She also called my father's doctor, a hypertension specialist at a major medical center in Manhattan, to alert him that my father was on his way.

My brother drove my father to the hospital, where his doctor ordered several tests, including an MRI. By now it was 5:00 P.M. My mother called to tell me that she was at the hospital with my brother and would phone me later.

The MRI showed that my father had suffered a mild stroke. But you know how it goes in hospitals: you wait, and you wait, and you wait some more. Finally, after waiting more than five hours, the hospital found him a bed. It was now almost 11:00 P.M. My father asked my brother to take him to the men's room, where he had another stroke, a massive one, and collapsed on the floor. It was the last time he would ever stand on his own two feet.

What happened? Could the second stroke have been prevented? Why was the doctor so nonchalant about my father's condition?

I know now that the high level of abnormal brain activity following a stroke makes people extremely vulnerable to additional strokes. Why did my father have to wait so long to be treated? Why wasn't he put on heparin? Was this a case of gross negligence, of malpractice?

We thought about bringing a lawsuit against the hospital, but we never did. My brother was advised that it would be very difficult to find doctors to testify as expert witnesses on our behalf. Also, our energies were consumed by the crisis of the present and our fears for the future.

Of the regrets I have about what I did or did not do during my father's stroke, I do not regret my wish not to sue. What would have been the point? My father was paralyzed, and no amount of money would have changed that and restored him to health.

When I visit my father the day after his stroke, I am stunned. He is strapped to a flat metal slab in a cubicle of the hospital ICU. He is not in a bed, as I had expected. There is someone else in the room, standing near the bed, crying softly: my mother. But I have eyes only for my father. When I last saw him, two weeks ago, his sparse circle of hair was gray. Now it is completely white. Even worse is the sight of his immobilized body beneath the sheet that covers him. He looks like the hulk of a ship. My mother leans over and whispers to me that when she saw my father, she nearly fainted.

Every few minutes a nurse comes in and checks his pulse or his blood pressure. "You know, your father is quite a charmer," she says cheerfully. "He's had all of us laughing." Oh, really? I have to admit there is something comfortingly familiar about that.

"They keep asking me who the president is," says a garbled voice I've never heard before, a voice that comes from my father. "Of course I know who the president is," says the mangled voice. My head begins to spin. "Yes, Dad," I say, my lips pulled back to form a smile. Perhaps this is what is expected of me, to keep things light, to pretend this is a joke. "Of course you know who the president is." I stumble out of the ICU into the waiting room, where I am told my father's doctors want to speak with me.

By the time the three men in white coats step off the elevator and approach me, I can no longer feel my body. My hands: are they still attached to my arms? I feel as if I am dissolving—literally melting—and I wonder whether the doctors can see this or if I am the only one who knows. Besides, are there really three of them, or is there just one and I'm having hallucinations? Why do they look exactly alike? And what is this they are saying? Condition very serious. First twenty-four hours critical. Possibility of cerebral hemorrhage. Not sure of the extent of damage.

I begin to sense their heads bobbing up and down like a chorus of puppets and my head starts to bob up and down in unison with theirs. Suddenly I have a vision of the four of us standing there in the waiting room, our heads bobbing up and down together, and I nearly laugh out loud. "Thank you, thank you for taking such good care of him," I hear myself say while my hand shoots out to meet theirs.

Like a fleet of small boats, they turn away and enter the elevator. I stand and watch while the gray metal doors close slowly in front of them.

Of my father's many losses after the stroke, I mourned tennis first. When I was in college, I came home one summer and told him that I had met a young man whom I liked very much, and that things had gotten pretty serious between us. The first question my father asked was, "Is he Jewish?" The second was, "Does he play tennis?"

My father was rather comical-looking on the tennis court. Short and bald, with his paunch bulging through his white Lacoste shirt. His shorts were baggy and wrinkled. On his head he wore a squashed terry cloth hat to protect his scalp from the sun. He was bowlegged and scrambled across the court like a crab. His strokes were awkward. However, he had never lost the fierce determination of his youth, which earned him the nickname "the scrapper" from my husband. He frequently called his opponents' shots out when they were not. He was famous for these line calls; three people who spoke at his funeral mentioned them. But he was also funny, friendly, and generous to his friends, qualities that endeared him to many.

When I take my son for afternoon tennis lessons in the months after the stroke, I see a group of older men playing doubles. I stare at these grandfathers while they amiably lob balls back and forth, ribbing each other and laughing. I cannot accept that my father will never do this again. As they saunter off the court, I want to rush up to them, shake them, and scream, "You have no idea how lucky you are. No idea!"

But maybe they do know they are lucky. After all, they are about the same age as my father. As I watch them put on their jackets, I grieve for my father lying paralyzed in a hospital bed.

Over the next few days following my father's stroke I develop a new routine: wake up, get the kids to school, cry, go to the hospital, cry, come home, get dinner ready, help the kids with their homework, get them ready for bed, cry, go to sleep.

Before my father's stroke, I had been studying for the qualifying exams for my doctorate in English. Now I can't study. I am too tired to concentrate, and the words in my books are incomprehensible, slithering about meaninglessly on the page. So I put my texts aside and carry around my stroke notebook instead.

My father spent three months in institutions: two weeks in the hospital, six weeks at a sub-acute rehab facility, and four weeks in the acute rehab unit at Kessler. This is an unusual progression, to go from sub-acute rehab to acute – it usually works the other way around – but Kessler's acute unit kept rejecting my father. After weeks of relenting, pleading, and, finally, an on site evaluation, Kessler accepted him. I was overjoyed. Kessler is known throughout the world. I thought surely they could fix my father, help him learn to walk again. But on his last day at Kessler his doctor apologizes, saying the paralysis is too dense. There will be no return of mobility in his paralyzed arm or leg. My father will be confined to a wheelchair the rest of his life.

My father lived at home for five years. Five years of loss: the loss of independence, the activities that gave him pleasure – tennis, bridge, movies, concerts, traveling – the loss of his identity as a provider, the loss of his role as an able-bodied companion and spouse, the loss of his ability to play with his grandchildren. It's not just the wheelchair. After the stroke my father's diabetes went out of control. His short-term memory was compromised. He was weak and easily fatigued.

He was a very sick man.

Then my father loses his battle against diabetes. One day the podiatrist gives him the terrible news: he has gangrene.

I thought gangrene died with the soldiers of World War I. People don't expire from gangrene anymore—this is the beginning of the new millennium. But new millennium or not, my father has gangrene and is going to lose his left leg.

My father does not want to have his leg amputated. He says he would rather die of the infection. "Let me die," he says to us.

The doctor tells him that gangrene is a gruesome death. It is slow and excruciating, even with morphine. It can take months to die of gangrene. "The body putrefies," the nurses whisper to my mother. "The stench is awful."

All right, dying of gangrene is not an option. The amputation is scheduled.

My father's leg is amputated on July 20, 2000, my forty-fourth birthday. On the way to the hospital the day of the surgery my car is rear-ended at the entrance to Route 46. I jump out of my out and start yelling at the shaken young woman who hit me. "My father is having his leg amputated today," I feel like screaming.

At the hospital, my father is in great pain, moaning and thrashing. He cannot take painkillers before the operation.

The minutes tick slowly by as my mother and I wait for the attendants to get him. As soon as they place him on the gurney, I rush out of the room, get in my car, and race for home. I plan to come back tomorrow. I do not have the courage to be there when my father returns without his left leg.

After the amputation I have nightmares about the missing limb.

"What happens to amputated limbs?" I ask my husband. He says they are disposed of with the medical waste.

The thought of my father's leg being dumped in the garbage is too much. I have visions of finding it and bringing it back to life. When I go to the hospital to visit, I cannot rid myself of the idea that the leg is inside a closet, waiting for me to resuscitate it.

My father stops speaking after the amputation. He will answer a question with a monosyllable, but that's it. I recently found a letter dated July 23, 2000, that I wrote but never sent:

> *Dear Dad,*
>
> *I am writing to you because every time I see you I am filled with emotion and find it hard to express my feelings. We are all very sorry for this terrible thing that has befallen you. We know you are suffering. None of us will ever know how much.*
>
> *That said, we also suffer. The world isn't black and white. Although we can't feel your pain, that doesn't mean we feel no pain.*
>
> *We cannot bring back to you what you have lost but we still have something to give you—our deep, abiding love. You are still the head of our family. I am begging you to try to come to terms with this loss. We are here for you; please don't turn us away.*
>
> *Your loving daughter,*
>
> *Nancy*

I don't regret not sending this letter. What difference would it have made?

I should have sent the letter.

Two months after the amputation, my father goes into Northridge Manor Nursing Home. The aide can't get him out of bed. He does not have the strength to help with transfers from the bed to the wheelchair. It takes two very strong people to lift him, and my mother's osteoporosis means she is not able to assist.

Northridge Manor looks something like a hotel. The halls are papered in a cheerful red-and-white chrysanthemum pattern, with deep green carpeting to match. If you close your eyes to the people in wheelchairs and the nurses at their stations, you might pretend you are in a Hilton. There is even a tiny coffee shop with a few scattered bistro tables and chairs.

My father likes to be taken to the coffee shop for ice cream floats, which are made with sugar-free ice cream and Diet Coke for diabetic patients like him. He can make that drink last for a good half hour. These outings for ice cream make our visits easier for me, because they give us something to do.

When I visit the nursing home, I arrive buoyed by a sense of mission and purpose: I am here to do a *mitzvah,* a good deed: to spend time with my sick father. I am cheered by the silk flowers on the lobby table and the announcement of the week's activities on the bulletin board. "This isn't such a bad place," I say.

But by the time I reach his floor, I am shaken. There is no use pretending that this is some kind of vacation spot. In the dayroom men and women doze in their metal chairs. From one of the rooms a woman's voice keeps crying, "Nurse, Nurse!" Beneath the sickly sweet smell of antiseptic wafts another odor—familiar, unpleasant, soiled.

My father's room is at the end of a long corridor. Usually he is sleeping when I arrive. A private-duty aide hired by my mother sits in a chair, reading or watching television.

Sometimes he opens his eyes and says, "Hi, *schaetzle.*" Sometimes he doesn't respond until the aide nudges his shoulder and says, "Charlie, Charlie. Nancy is here."

During these visits I try to assume an air of bravado, thinking maybe I can cheer or distract him. Any subject I can think of—my children, sports, current events, even the weather—especially the weather, since he rarely goes outside—only deepens the chasm between us. I am part of a busy, active world and my father is not.

I also suspect he is angry with me because he thinks I have betrayed him. I participated in the family conspiracy that put him in this awful place.

I feel guilty all the time.

The women in my support group agree we always feel guilty. Guilty that we aren't always available for our parents. Guilty that we sometimes feel angry with them. Guilty that we want our own lives. Guilty that we can't change anything.

Guilty that we are healthy and they are not.

The group facilitator would ask us, "Do you think this guilt is productive? Does it help you become better caregivers?"

We knew the answer to these questions was "no," but we felt guilty anyway.

The smell of the nursing home is something else. There is an odor of disinfectant masking the smell of human waste. I try not to breathe through my nose when I visit, which means that by the time I leave, I have a terrible headache.

The halls are scrupulously clean, so it's not that the place looks dirty. No, the soiling is elsewhere. It's written on faces, bodies like mashed fruit. Women with red and purple bruises on their arms and legs. Women with hair as fine as gossamer silk and smiles as sad as a goodbye kiss. Men babbling or groaning. Men in the halls thrusting their shriveled arms in my face. "Won't you fix my footrest, miss? Please, please, won't you help me?"

I try not to look or listen. I walk down the corridors rapidly, my eyes focused forward, my thoughts focused inward. I must minimize what I feel. I have my own deep sorrows to contend with. I cannot help these people.

My father has been a resident of Northridge Manor for about nine months when suddenly he becomes very ill. Out of the blue, he spikes a fever of 103; he is delirious and sent to the hospital. The doctors determine that the fever is caused by a staph infection; after a few days of testing, they discover he has sepsis, which cannot be treated with antibiotics and is fatal.

After consulting with the doctors, my father is taken off anything that would sustain life: food, water, insulin, all medications. Even so, he lingers.

It is absolutely wrenching to watch a loved one die. At the end, after all the years of planning, coping, and managing my father's illness, things fall apart. We do not make visitation schedules. Sometimes my mother, brother, and I are there together in my father's room, sometimes one of us is there—sometimes, no one is there. The hours and days creep slowly by.

There is nothing we can do. At first my father is restless and moans, but then he is too weak to do anything. A nurse comes in periodically and adjusts the level of morphine in his IV. Or she gives us washcloths and cups of chipped ice so we can wipe his lips, which are dry and cracked. He is not unconscious, but he is too exhausted to speak. It is not a beautiful death.

How did we get the idea that death should be beautiful? Maybe from nineteenth-century sentimental novels, where the family gathers around the deathbed of the loved one, who is gazing beatifically toward the heavens and saying things like, "I'm ready now."

The days somehow pass. Word has spread that my father is dying and people come to pay their respects. A few hold his hand as they whisper good-bye. My father doesn't open his eyes.

One of my father's tennis buddies, a rabbi who had supervised the synagogue religious school when I was a student there, comes to say farewell. "It's time, Charlie," he says, taking my father's hand. "You can let go now." I hold my breath. "Oh my God," I think. "This is it. It's going to happen, and I'm going to be the only one here from my family." But nothing happens.

The doctors tell us that if he hangs on for more than a week, he will be transferred back to the nursing home. I pray that won't happen.

On the day that turns out to be the last, I find myself at the hospital at about 6:00 in the evening. My brother and mother have been there since early morning. I tell them to go home and rest, then I take a seat next to his bed.

I pull my chair over to his bed and lift his hand, which is thin and translucent as an onion's skin. "Dad," I say. "Do you know who this is?"

Silence.

"Dad," I press on. "Say my name."

Silence. I am in turmoil, angry at myself for making demands of a dying man, angry at him for what feels like stubbornness.

"Dad, I know you're in there."

Silence. I am about to give up when, out of the blue, I hear, "Nancy."

I am overjoyed that he has made contact. I move even closer and bend my head to meet his. I want desperately to maintain the connection. I can think of nothing meaningful to tell him so I say, "This isn't easy, is it?" And my father whispers, "Nothing is easy."

And then, silence. I know that this silence will be the longest one, that my father will not speak to me again.

And indeed, those are the last words I hear. That evening, shortly after midnight, my father slips into a coma and passes away. We are not there to send him off.

He dies alone.

When I think back to that evening, I try to recall if I knew it would be his last. I try to remember whether the night nurse, who watched me leave at 9:00 P.M., raised her eyebrows as if to ask me where did I think I was going. These are the traces of guilt playing tricks with my imagination. The nurses see all kinds of families and all kinds of deaths. Throughout my father's days, they were efficient and professional. They tried to relieve my father's suffering but they did not offer advice or sympathy, which was a great relief. If they judge the actions of the living, they have the decency to keep their opinions to themselves.

There was no deathbed scene, no family gathering, no hand-holding, no chanting of prayers or hymns. When I tell this to an acquaintance, she is horrified. She tells me the story of how her family helped her father leave this world. They kept vigil for hours, she says, for days, even. When I talk about how unbearable it was at the end, how, ultimately, none of us could stand to watch the suffering anymore, another friend says she still feels guilty that she wasn't with her mother when her mother passed away.

There is no proper way to die, and there are no rules. We must all live with our own consciences and we have no authority to declare to our fellow travelers, "You should have done this, or done that."

My father died in the early morning hours of Tuesday, June 19, 2001. He was buried the next day. According to Jewish law, burial should take place as quickly as possible, although not during the Sabbath. Custom dictates that the deceased be buried in a plain pine coffin (always closed during the service) and mourned for seven days.

For years Jews have fiddled with these traditions. My father was buried in a walnut coffin—a little more elegant—and my mother sat *shivah* for three days. There are other rules governing cremation, which is forbidden in Jewish law, and the donation of organs for research or transplantation, verboten as well. I know Jewish families who have ignored these prohibitions. But I have never seen an open coffin at a Jewish funeral.

I think the chapel at the funeral home was full. It seemed as though a few hundred people filled the pews. The rabbi had told me that he would lead a brief service and then ask my brother and I to speak.

I sat in the front pew and stared straight ahead, trying hard not to lose my composure. The rabbi must have noticed my effort, because he changed the order of speakers and asked me to speak first, before my brother. I was grateful for his sensitivity because I was rapidly losing my grip.

Giving a eulogy in front of that crowd of people was one of the most difficult challenges I've ever faced. I had prepared a brief text, in which I tried to capture my father's spirit:

"As you know, my father was a CPA, an accountant. But his personality did not go with the job description. He was far more interested in people than in debits and credits. He had a wonderful sense of humor, and even when he was very ill he could still make people laugh. I know that he would be pleased that so many dear friends and family have come today to honor him."

"Friendship mattered a great deal to him. Some of his friendships went back over fifty years, to his early days as an immigrant to this country. He made friends from many avenues and interests: UJA, B'nai B'rith, the synagogue, tennis, bridge, work. When my father liked you, he liked you for life."

"My father was a tenacious man. If you'd ever played tennis with him, you'd know what I mean. He chased down every ball as though his life depended on it. Out of respect for his memory, I will say nothing about his line calls."

"My father's last words were, 'Nothing is easy.' I think they testify to his fighting spirit, his tenacity. I think he was trying to tell me that a life well lived requires hard work. He worked hard all his life, and most especially when he was ill. He has earned this final rest."

I rested my hand on the coffin as I left the podium to return to my seat. It flashed through my mind that the gesture might appear theatrical, but I didn't care. This was my final chance to say good-bye.

My brother talked about Aaron Copeland's "Fanfare for the Common Man" and how it reminded him of my father: heroic, triumphant, accessible.

My mother read a selection from Ecclesiastes, known to the children of the sixties as a protest song by The Byrds: "To Everything Turn, Turn, Turn."

After that, memory blurs. Several other people spoke, and most of them mentioned my father's infamous line calls, where the opponent's ball was always out. I'm not sure whether he would have found that funny.

When my father still lived at home, he told me he wished for two things: to see my son become Bar Mitzvah, and to see me complete my doctorate in English.

My son became Bar Mitzvah on October 18, 1998.

My father could not go up to the *bima,* the synagogue pulpit, for his *aliyah* because it was not wheelchair accessible. The rabbi brought the Torah to him. I will never forget watching him touch the fringes of his *tallit,* the prayer shawl, to his lips and then to the Torah, the traditional gesture of kissing the sacred scroll, and the sound of his gravelled voice chanting the blessings before and after the *parsha,* the portion. Later I heard that throughout the sanctuary people were weeping. My father had been practicing the *brachot,* the blessings, for weeks.

In October 1999 I completed my doctorate from Rutgers. My father was too weak to attend the ceremony.

Years have passed since my father died, and I often ruminate on the stroke.

One day I went looking through my father's business diaries. My father was not much of a correspondent so I have no letters from him. I had not known he'd kept a diary of sorts, so the stash of volumes satisfied my need to have something he'd written.

The diaries record the full life of a busy man. They are handsome books, chestnut leather with an alligator pattern. He received them as yearly Christmas gifts from a company from which he purchased insurance against credit card fraud. I guess such insurance was inexpensive and worth the peace of mind. I tried to contact the company and order but a Google search told me the firm had gone bankrupt.

Tucked inside the diary for 1995—the year he had the stroke, and the last one he kept -- were all kinds of papers: receipts for plumbing and heating maintenance; business cards from electricians and repair contractors; strips of paper with names and phone numbers of bridge and tennis partners; concert programs; a brochure for East Hampton House, a hotel where he and my mother spent a long weekend a month before the stroke.

Each day contains a few mere jottings. Here's a typical entry: "Odds and ends. Finished McAllister payroll taxes. Unity Concerts." Or, "Lunch with Eli and the boys at the diner. Movies with Trudy; saw 'Nobody's Fool.'" Or, on a Sunday: "Larry here; watched Browns v. New England."

He also documented the weather: "Hot and humid." "Beautiful day, 70 degrees." The entry for Friday, February 24, 1995: "Cool today. Great bridge. Nancy attacked."

I was attacked, mugged one night by a stranger who sneaked up behind my back, hit me on the head with his fist, and ran off with my purse while I was trying to unlock my kitchen door. I had forgotten the date. It's curious to me that my father noted it in the same detached tone he used to record watching a football game. On the other hand, in the shock of reading those words, "Nancy attacked," I hear the echoes of his own distress.

Sometimes I ask myself what I learned from my father's illness.

I've learned to slow down a bit. I've learned to be less afraid of speaking my mind. I've learned about my own ageism. I'm still learning.

What did my father learn, if anything, from his illness?

That is a more complicated question. He never spoke to me directly of how his understanding of himself changed. He had moved quite suddenly from a place of privilege and dominance within our family to one of powerlessness and invisibility. Even though my life revolved around the stroke for six years, the demands of his illness drove my actions and emotions, rather than my dealings with him and the new person he had become.

I regret that I was not able to get to know my new father.

I took his silences as an accusation; I never understood that what he wanted was companionship, not entertainment. I didn't have to try so hard.

On Rosh Hashanah, the start of the new Jewish year, I'll visit your grave, with its granite headstone the color of fresh earth. I'll place a small rock on top to mark my visit. I'll utter a prayer for refuah sh'lamah, peace and healing in the world. We need that right now. Those are things you would have wanted, too.

It's time to lay my pen to rest.

Brad Saul vs. Multiple Sclerosis:
Grit, Determination and Kindness
by Pierre C. Bouvard

I met Brad Saul in 1980 at Northwestern University when he was a graduate student chosen by the School of Communication to oversee the student radio station. I was the sophomore General Manager.

The Brad I met that year clearly lived the Steve Job's sentiment of "Find what you love, and love what you do". Brad was the constant entrepreneur to whom the solution to the problem was a business. He was the consummate sales person who lived the mantra of "always be closing".

Love for AM/FM Radio Made Us Brothers

For Brad and I, it was radio love at first sight. I had interned and worked at radio stations in Boston and Chicago. Brad was a radio rock star. By the tender age of 20, he had already worked at CBS's WBBM-AM in Chicago and had worked as General Managers of two radios stations all while going to Northwestern.

Brad and I loved talking about radio, sales and business ideas. He had a good sense of humor and we would regale each other with stories and impersonations. He was a force of nature, overflowing with ideas.

The spark of his love for radio was forged in the early 70's when he was attending an Evanston Street Fair with his parents. WLTD-AM Evanston's Chuck Schaden was broadcasting "Those Were The Days," a retro show that instantly made a momentous impression on 13-year-old Brad. Soon Brad was on the air on Schaden's Saturday morning show called `Radio For Kids,' which featured a different weekly co-host. Brad told radio trade publication Inside Radio "That was my first on-air radio thing. I still have the script where I read the first weather forecast I ever did on the air."

Not only did the radio spark light up, but so did Brad's amazing entrepreneurial talent.

Witnessing Schaden on that Saturday event prompted Brad to sell copies of old radio shows. Brad bought an ad in a physician's journal. Why physicians journals? Richard, his stepfather, is a physician.

Brad was flooded with orders for copies of the old radio shows. At the time, there was no such thing as high-speed duplication. The duplication consisted of making copies from one cassette recorder to another in his bedroom. Operations had to be suspended because the young Brad literally had too much business.

Flash forward to college, Brad is in his freshman year at the University of Missouri, and then WWBM-AM Chicago came calling. WBBM 780 AM was Chicago's all news radio station.

Brad said "I couldn't quit college because guilt would be with me forever, So I applied to the one school, Northwestern University, I was absolutely sure I wouldn't get into." From 400 applications that year, Northwestern accepted seven transfer students – including Brad - who claims the only reason he was chosen was that the Dean of Students liked him.

Brad was ever resourceful. To subsidize his education, Brad used his Spanish-language fluency to hold a number of jobs, including acting as a Spanish talk show host. Brad said, "I did whatever I could do, including donating blood, It came with a free meal, orange juice and cookies. I ate peanut butter and crackers six nights a week and cauliflower the seventh because I needed a vegetable."

Love What You Do, Do What You Love

Along the way, Brad ran WEEF-AM Highland Park, IL. Brad had me come up to the station and pre- recorded station ID's that say the name of the station and explains what the station's goal. Brad's powers of persuasion were impressive.

Here I am, a catholic kid from Massachusetts booming out "WEEF 1430 AM, We're all things Jewish!!!" What does it mean to be all things Jewish?? I had no idea! But if you listened to WEEF AM 1430 in Highland Park you could find out!!!

I remember that AM radio station in Evanston where Brad first caught the radio bug. Brad became its General Manager, and he turned the station from a money-losing Beautiful Music format into a successful Spanish station.

When Brad was a sophomore, a new soccer team came to Chicago. Knowing that soccer is very popular in the Spanish community, Brad wanted to secure the Spanish radio rights for his station and the owner of the team said to Brad, "let's go out for dinner with my wife and I and you and your lady." The problem was that Brad was a sophomore in college and trying to appear like someone much older. It would not work to take a Northwestern girl who would give Brad's real age away. The ever resourceful Brad pressed his beloved cousin Betsy into service. Betsy was already in the working world as a finance professional and would fit the role. The dinner went very well. The awkward moment came when the team owner asked Brad and Betsy how they met. They both blurted out at the same time: blind date! Met at a party! They corrected each other, blind date at a party!

Turning Problems into Solutions

Now we come to the genius of Brad. Here is how he turns a problem into a solution, and create a business. As a radio station General Manager, Brad recognized the challenges faced by local stations to provide quality public service programming. According to FCC regulations, every local station had to identify problems and issues in their market and then create programming to discuss the issues. This was difficult for local stations. Having to create unique programming to address these local issues, find the appropriate guests and then produce the show.

Brad's brilliant solution was to create public service programming that many stations could use as their own. Brad knew that in Chicago, he could produce better programming for the stations, and offer them on a barter basis. Barter means that stations get free programming in exchange for airing commercials. Brad's first company, Public Interest Affiliates, was born.

In the 60's and 70's airlines paid for in flight music and audio to entertain air travelers. Following deregulation in 1981, airlines no longer wanted to pay for such programming.

It occurred to Brad there were similarities between in-flight programming and bartered syndication. Once again, there was a Brad Saul master stroke. He provided the airlines with free in-flight audio and video programming in exchange for running advertising.

Eastern became the first airline to allow Public Interest Affiliates to sell in-flight audio commercials on a barter basis. It was so successful, that Eastern asked Brad and his company to do the same for their in-flight television programming. Soon Brad's company was doing in-flight programming and ad sales for American, Eastern, TWA, United and Western.

Barbara Nelson, who was part of Public Interest Affiliates in 1980's told me,

Brad's company, has and always will hold a special place in my heart as I've never worked with a more fun, dynamic and hilarious group of people. Brad was the utmost entrepreneur and never stopped trying, thinking or creating.

Realizing that the NBA was the only professional sports league without a network radio deal, Saul convinced the league to use his firm to create the NBA Radio Network in 1989.

All of these amazing professional accomplishments occurred before Brad Saul had turned 30. By the way, during all of this, Brad completed an undergraduate and a graduate degree in Radio, TV and Film at Northwestern , as well as a law degree at Loyola!

At the NBA pitch, Brad was captivated by an NBA employee, Debbie, and the two fell in love.

Europe 1989: The Best Trip We Ever Took

Two years before his diagnosis, Brad and I took a wonderful European trip. We spent time with my parents in the South of France and in the French Alps, and we stopped in London, Paris and Geneva. Each day we would enjoy breakfast and pour over newspapers. We would discuss the business news and consider the implications of the trends we read. We had become like twin brothers.

Multiple Sclerosis at 30 Years Old

In 1991, Brad was diagnosed with Multiple Sclerosis, but Brad and Debbie courageously agreed to move forward with their marriage. Brad told an industry trade publication in 2006, *"She is the most wonderful thing that ever happened to me!"*

After much effort, in 1999, Brad and Debbie welcomed triplets Gabrielle, Griffen and Brennan into their family.

Brad began to have difficulty walking and his experience with his disability make him realize he needed to help others to learn the business he loved so much. The ever-resourceful Brad established the Radio Center for People With Disabilities to recruit, train and place people with disabilities into radio station jobs.

A three hour wait in his wheelchair for a ride in a snowstorm was Brad's next inspiration. There were so few taxis that could accommodate people with physical challenges. To Brad, the solution to the problem is a business. With the help of Yellow Cab Chicago owner Pat Corrigan, Brad established Chicago Disability Transit. The objective was to create more vehicles that could transport people with physical challenges to and from medical facilities and around Chicago.

Brad was the ultimate sales person. There's a line in the movie Glengarry Glen Ross about sales, "Always be Closing". In other words, ask for the order.

Just one month before his death in December 2015. Brad was in a medical facility and he asked the staff whom they used for transportation. It turns out they were highly dissatisfied with their current provider. A few days later, Brad was out of the facility and made a personal sales call. He got the deal for Chicago Disability Transit. He called me because he was so excited, so proud.

Brad Meant the World to Me

At two crucial moments in my life he literally saved me. One time there was a women who was wrong for me and I knew it. But I felt an obligation to proceed with the relationship, marriage and to be there for her six year old boy. Brad made sure I made the right decision. He was relentless insisting that I made the right decision.

The next time it was a big life changing job offer. I was torn because I liked so much what I was doing that I couldn't decide. It took Brad a month of nightly phone calls to get me to make the right decision. Brad said he got grey hair trying to help through that decision.

Jeff Smulyen, the CEO of Emmis Communications, one of America's most respected radio broadcasting groups, loved Brad. Hearing of Brad's failing health, he dropped everything in November of 2015 and drove four hours from Indianapolis to sit with Brad. It meant the world to Brad.

The Pain and Agony of a Disease

Brad used his stunning intelligence, grit and resourcefulness to attack MS with full force. He read voraciously about the disease, the new cures in trial and new medications. He amazed his doctors with his knowledge, intelligence and determination to try the next solution and the next.

Since I lived in New York City, we would talk for hours on the telephone. I learned that Brad would investigate technologies that allowed him to dictate his sales letters and proposals. One of the greatest joys he experienced was wearing a device called an exoskeleton.

This was an amazing machine that allowed people with disabilities to walk. The suit returns movement to wearers' hips and knees with small motors attached to standard orthotics. Wearers can control the movement of each leg and walk at up to 1.1 miles per hour by pushing buttons integrated into a pair of crutches. A battery pack worn as a backpack powers the exoskeleton for up to eight hours. Brad could not afford the device, but dreamed of having it so he could walk again. The loss of his mobility and the realization that his health was deteriorating was depressing to Brad. He wrote a close friend:

> *"I just had this really morbid thought.*
>
> *If I had died years ago when I was at the top of my game, I don't know how many people would have remembered me, but I would have been remembered.*
>
> *If I die now/tomorrow, I don't think anybody would remember me.*
>
> *I really don't know that I have done anything that is memorable for them (the kids).*
>
> *I know I'm not alone. There are certainly a lot of people that were at the top of whatever they did, and for lots of other reasons went quietly into that good night. Barely a memory for anyone.*
>
> *It's like I said to you in my message. A year ago today I found a way out for myself. Walking in the exoskeleton is something I will never forget.*
>
> *At the same time, I can never forget all of I have lost in the year since."*

Roberta Grimes is a host on Brad's WebTalkRadio.net podcasting platform who speaks about death and the afterlife. She wrote:

> *Brad and I talked often and at length about his frustrations with his health and what death would be like for him. I gave him as a gift, a reading with an*

extraordinary spiritual medium. The spiritual medium sent Roberta an email this morning and said she just saw a man she thought was Brad stand up from his wheelchair and wave his arms in a big "Ta-da!" Roberta says, "He has a healthy young body now in a beautiful place, like earth-perfection magnified; he couldn't continue to live here as he was. I hope that comforts you, dear friends. I find that it helps a little. But I just really miss him!

Gabby, Griffen and Brennan: the Love of Brad's Life

Brad was bursting with pride in 2013 when his children had their bar and bat- mitzvah. When asked by the Chicago Tribune was his fantasy was, Brad said, *to be able to play baseball with my kids. Right now, because of multiple sclerosis, I can't walk, much less run.*

I told Brad that being a dad is not just throwing a ball. But more importantly it's being there, listening to them, sharing your wisdom, and giving them ideas. The traits of Brad's kindness, gifts, and curiosity live on in his children. Over the last 16 years, he told me countless stories of how proud he was of his kids. He regaled me with tales of their talents and gifts. Gabby, was a good writer and wonderful dancer. Brennan and Griffen were good athletes and did well in school. A week before he died, Brad showed me the parent portal at the schools and beamed with pride over the amazing grades in challenging courses.

A month before Brad died, Brad's son Griffen made an amazing speech in honor of his father at his school which is posted on YouTube. Griffen has started an organization to help people with Disabilities in honor of his dad.

In his speech, Griffen said:

"You either define your faith, or you are defined by it.

There are certain moments in every persons life, where we have to make a choice. Will we succumb to challenges, or will we persevere, and become the person that we want to be. There is no better representation that this than my father Brad Saul. My father has such a strong heart and will to live, that he was able to fight his way back through months of therapy. Unfortunately he had only won a single battle. The war had just begun.

Since then he has been in and out of the hospital. We live every day to the fullest.

My dad has shocked doctors with his ability to fight. But I am afraid his will to keep fighting is just running out. It is so painful to watch someone you love go through such unimaginable suffering. I could let my emotional struggle define me or I use those challenges and turn them into positive, something that would help me and change the world and become the person that I would want to be.

I found that I was able to connect with them in ways that others could not, due to my fathers disabilities. It was during my freshman year, when my dad fell ill, that I had been able to realize my dream, to start my own non- profit organization, with the mission being to empower youth with disabilities and their families to better improve the quality of their lives. The dream was to make sure that no person or no family would ever have to go through the emotional pain that my family and I had to go through."

Craig Killberger, and Free the Children inspired Griffen to "Make a change". An email from Craign Killbeerger told Griffen:

I believe that we can each create positive change by using a simple equation, issue plus gift equals better world. An issue is something that sparks your interest, something that you saw is wrong and decided to do something about it. Something that has impacted your world, such as multiple sclerosis.

The second part of your equation. Your gift is also critical. Everyone has a gift. For some people their gift is compassion. They have the innate ability to listen to others and offer empathy. Griffen I believe that you have those gifts.

> *It is the people who no one imagines anything of, that do the things that no one can imagine.*

Griffen's has three simple requests.

- *Take initiative and never be afraid to request help.*

- *We have all suffered pain and loss. Yet that does not make us who we are. We all have the ability to do something amazing.*

- *Be the change that you want to see in the world. Everyone has a gift, put effort to define what it is. We are the next generation of change. We are the problem solvers. Everyone of you will change the world.*

Koysta, Zibbie, Raoul and Jay: the Care Givers

In Brad's remaining years, he needed caregivers to help him get cleaned, dressed and get ready for the day. His parents generously supported the care givers.

Each of them were kind, gentle and patient, feeding him, brushing his hair and picking up objects, acts that most people can do for themselves, but Brad needed help. They were there every step of the way to help him at night, in the morning and during the day.

One of the best memories I had with Brad was a warm summer in 2014, the Chicago Air Show had jets soaring over Lake Michigan. Brad waved off his anxious care takers and we went down by the shore. We smoked cigars and took in the amazing views.

2015: A Difficult Last Year

The last half of 2014 and 2015 was challenging for Brad. He spent a number of months in and out of the hospital, with surgeries and stays at rehabilitation facilities.

Brad was in the hospital in late September when I visited him. One of Brad's businesses was his WebTalkRadio web site, where authors and experts hosted short radio shows or podcasts.

I was stunned to see Brad in the hospital and on the phone providing coaching to one of his hosts. The phone was positioned so Brad could speak to his host without using his hands.

On October 30th, 2015 Brad sent me an email:

> *We need to find some time to talk this weekend. I am over in the hospital, but my circumstances have changed. Debbie and I have decided that I want to be in Palliative care. I do not want to keep rolling into and out the hospital every few weeks. I want to be at home with my family and in a loving environment. Eating smarter with better food choices will also help keep me out of the hospital. I just spent another six weeks there, and all of May. This does not mean I am giving up, or that I am going to die. So are you in over the weekend?*

Debbie contacted me November 28th 2015 and said that things were touch and go with Brad. I flew to Chicago to find Brad very thin, tired and having a hard time breathing.

One of Brad's most cherished professional colleagues was Emmis Radio CEO Jeff Smulyan. Jeff is one of the smartest and nicest people in the radio business. Years ago, he and Brad had struck up a friendship that continued over the years with lengthy phone calls and emails, and sharing bat and bar mitzvahs.

Jeff and I were in constant contact about Brad, and he implored me to keep him up to date on the state of Brad's health. Despite all the pressures and demands of running a public radio company and spearheading the innovation NextRadio FM listening smartphone app, Jeff asked that I call him as soon as I landed in Chicago on that cold November Sunday night.

I spoke to Jeff as soon I arrived that night, and told Jeff that Debbie said it was not clear how long Brad had. Jeff literally dropped everything and got in his car and drove to Chicago from Indianapolis that evening.

To say Brad was elated to see Jeff walk through the door was an understatement. For several hours, the three of us talked about the radio business and the media industry.

I contacted Tom Keramidas, one of our great friends from our Northwestern days. The next day Tom quickly came over to Brad and Debbie's apartment. It was clear Brad was so happy to see Tom once again. I was sitting with Brad by his bed, holding his hand, when my cell phone rang. It was my mom. Over the years she had been like a second mom to Brad. She was upset. She sensed Brad was not doing well and had a premonition that he had died.

I put the cell phone on speaker and she was able to say some sweet and kind words to Brad, and she repeated what she always said to him, that he was an easy pregnancy for her. He had a hard time speaking, but I told my mom her words were heard and it meant a lot to Brad.

On the bureau near Brad was his wedding photo. The contrast between the happy, physically strong man, and the man in the bed was stunning. It seemed as if fifty years had passed.

On Tuesday December 1, 2015 I hugged Brad's slender frame for the last time. As I traveled back to New York, I had the comfort of knowing that Brad's most cherished cousin Betsy was coming in that day to spend the several days with Brad.

On December 4th Debbie texted: "Brad's starting to tire out. He's been sleeping quite a bit these past couple of days, and has been taking more frequent doses of morphine."

Later than evening, Betsy, Brad's beloved cousin, called to say Brad had died. Within the hour, Debbie texted, "Pierre, I know you spoke to Betsy. He died very peacefully."

In hindsight, my visit, and that of Tom Keramidas and Jeff Smulyan had been perfectly timed. Brad had been able to enjoy their company and trade stories. Or perhaps, Brad had said his goodbyes and he was ready.

The Jewish Warmth of Family, Friends and Life Celebrations

Brad's funeral was Monday December 7th. My wife, Mary and I were so touched by the warm traditions of the Jewish faith. We asked if we could bring some food and Debbie responded, "Thank you for the offer. There's already an army of people here doing that. You know Jews and food."

Each night that week Debbie and Brad's apartment was bursting full of people from their synagogue, the kids school and their family. Photos my dad had taken of Brad were on display in the living room.

Joy and warmth was in every nook and cranny of the apartment. I spied a group of Brad's children with their friends talking and enjoying people's company as tables overflowed with all sorts of food.

As I walked down the cold Chicago street back to my hotel, I thought, that's how to celebrate a life, with lots people enjoying each others company and sharing stories about an amazing man. Brad Saul was so full of life, bristling with ideas, selling up a storm, a true visionary.

Now, two years later, I am sure Brad would be overjoyed to know his three children are thriving at an amazing college or University, each with their gifts, talents and personalities which in part, are Brad's heritage they carry. As for me, it was like losing a brother who will always be an inspiration.

Faith
by Tara Coyote

Faith is a five-letter word that embodies the wisdom and power of all things sacred. While journeying with a life-threatening illness, it has supported me and also allowed me to break down when I needed to. Faith is the deeply rooted strength that has gotten me through the most challenging moments of my journey over the last five years. It is the raft that has carried me on the most turbulent river of life. Without my belief in my ability to transcend limitations during that time, I would have drowned in fear, worry, anger and grief.

Since 2012, there have been many trying changes in my life. I had a wonderful husband, a brilliant teenage son, and two beautiful teenage step-children. I was owner and operator of a Pilates and Gyrotonic studio with a large, clientele and lived in a house in Marin County, California. Then a very difficult situation arose between my husband and I which eventually undermined our relationship and left me depressed and angry. But I reached deep into my heart for a thread of faith to pull me through this crisis, and was surprised to find this thread leading me to deeply reconnect with horses. I had loved horses as a child and they would heal my life.

I sold my business and my house, my husband and I separated, and I moved three hours north to Nevada City, CA. The money from the sale of one of the pieces of Gyrotonic equipment allowed me to buy Comanche, my first horse. Comanche is a 15-year-old Spanish Mustang who was taken out of the wild when he was a yearling. Through my connection with Comanche, I realized a wish to help others heal with horses in the same manner that they had helped me. I became trained in Equine Facilitated Learning by Linda Kohanov, the best selling author of 'The Tao of Equus' (New World Library, 2001).

During this period of upheaval, I knew there was another life waiting for me; I just had to listen and a path would appear. Together with my magical horse Comanche, I was eventually guided to a gorgeous equine property. It was on this property that I was able to open a retreat center to help others transform their lives with horse medicine. If I hadn't believed in the power of faith, I wouldn't have the courage to make the bold leap of changing my life.

Months after this dramatic transition, in October 2013, my closest friend of nineteen years, Deb, was diagnosed with Acute Myeloid Leukemia. She was 44 years old. I immediately became one of her main caregivers with her mother and husband. I was with her throughout her whole twenty-two-month journey through illness and ultimately her death. It was a heartbreaking loss. To witness Deb die so young was shocking and made me turn to my faith to survive.

Six months later, another close friend and family member, Rowen, was diagnosed with Stage three Colin Cancer. She was 46 at the time of her diagnosis. I was stunned. It was inconceivable to me how both of my beloved friends could be affected by cancer at such young ages.

Then exactly a year after Deb died, I was diagnosed with Stage three Breast Cancer. This distressing event was more than shocking. One thing was clear, cancer had become a prominent teacher in my life.

Immediately after my diagnosis, I flung myself into research about the best protocols for healing. I had witnessed Deb follow the standard protocol of treatment, which was several rounds of chemotherapy and an eventual bone marrow transplant. I saw her transform from a 110-pound, petite and vibrant beauty, at the time of her diagnosis, to a 65-pound skeleton at her death.

The prescribed and standard route of treatment offered to me was four months of chemotherapy, surgery, and radiation. Since I had an advanced cancer diagnosis, the allopathic solution was to dose my body with heavy chemotherapy to kill any trace of cancer. The oncologist told me that the chemotherapy would most likely make me very ill and cause me to be hospitalized. There was even a chance that I could die from this treatment. I was also informed that this same kind of chemotherapy would not be given to an older person, as it would most certainly kill them. Also my immune system would be severely compromised by the chemotherapy. I was more than upset to hear this news. It was strangely ironic that I appreciated the raw honesty from the oncologist.

The way the different courses of treatment were described were: rounds of chemotherapy directed at the breast tumor, then If the rounds of chemo shrunk the tumor, the following treatment would be a lumpectomy and radiation to kill any remaining cancer cells, with possibly more chemotherapy. If the initial chemotherapy did not shrink the tumor, then, according to this course of treatment, I would need a mastectomy.

I was told that this course of treatment would take about a year. There were also multiple side effects to consider such as early menopause, nausea, mouth sores, loss of appetite, hair loss, chemo-brain, swollen hands and feet, digestive distress, sexual dysfunction, anxiety and depression, a destroyed immune system and so much more.

I had spent countless hours at the hospital during the many traumatic months of losing my dearest friend Deb. I knew that I should choose a different path for my healing, one that was in alignment with my body, mind, and soul. That led me to the decision to reject the conventional treatments and instead allow the cancer to heal through a natural healing protocol. I felt deep down that I would rather die a natural death from cancer than submit my body to the poison and agony of chemotherapy. This was my first act of faith, making the empowered choice to heal myself.

As I researched and chose healing protocols, my parents, my brother, and my son were very concerned by my decision to go against the prescribed course of chemotherapy, surgery, and radiation. In retrospect, seven months into the journey, having my family so upset was the most stressful part of my treatment decision. To have people that you love the most question, doubt and confront you during an already tough situation is agonizing. Moving through that disagreement made me stronger to face the rough waves to come.

I have found that it takes courage, as well as faith to choose a path in opposition to mainstream belief systems. That same courage has also served me to remain in alignment with what is authentically true for myself. I had many persistent questions in my head: was I right to deny standard protocols to heal my body? Did I trust natural medicines? Did I truly believe I could heal myself? Over time, I came to believe that I could heal myself the way nature intended!

Some doctors actually told me they can tell from their first meeting with cancer patients who will live and who will not. It's a certain fire in their eyes, a passion for life, and the stamina to overcome the hurdles and psychological mountains that a cancer journey encompasses.

As I battled the shadows of my mind, it became clear that the memory of seeing my closest friend die was a deep fear that I could face a similar fate. I had to find my own truth in the story. The first hurdle in this search was realizing that my story was different than Deb's. Since I was still grieving the loss of Deb only a year earlier, it took all the strength I had to realize that Deb had her own fate, one that was indeed different than my own. I was facing the choice of wanting to live or die. In fact, I felt that my life depended on this very important decision. I did not have to die the way Deb did.

As I found the will to live and choose my way of life, I began to have a new perspective and ask different types of questions. It occurred to me that there had to be some bizarre reason why two of my closest friends and I were affected by cancer in our mid-forties. There must be a plan hidden within this twisted story of cancer and young death. Once I separated my story from Deb's, I understood that there was indeed a purpose beyond my being afflicted with cancer. It included the understanding of the role of grief, not only in my life, but also in the lives of others and in our culture.

I was nearly paralyzed by the grief from the loss of my closest friend of twenty years. Then I realized that we are not taught how to process grief in our culture, and instead place our sadness in a hidden container, and pretend that we are fine after losing those we love. The usual business protocol is to provide just a week off from work when experiencing a serious loss in one's life. How can a week be enough time to heal such a traumatic loss?

I began to see the need for an outlet for people dealing with grief. I was trained to work with horses and people in a healing manner. I decided to combine the practices of equine assisted personal development with grief rituals. 'Grief Rituals with Horses' was born through passion and necessity. The ranch I own, 'Wind Horse Sanctuary' offers Equine Facilitated Learning. The goal is to help people work towards social intelligence, leadership and self-awareness. I believe that most of our communication is non-verbal and that horses have intuition, and are able to receive and share their emotions with people who are close to them. The people partaking in one of the programs will leave with skills to support them in their daily lives. I found that they have learned more effective ways of relating with others, to feel less stress and more peace, to live in the present moment and explore new avenues of creativity.

The 'Grief Rituals with Horses' daylong events were a great success and helped many people. Some of the participants reported that the daylong ritual completely and positively changed their life. I ended up offering eight different grief rituals within the course of a year, which allowed space for about 150 people to shed tears for their loved ones, pets, lost jobs, relationships, houses, the environment, and all the unexpressed sorrows they were carrying. I'm grateful that I was able to turn such a tragic event into a way to help others to express and heal their own grief. It was faith that helped me through the pain and that allowed something beautiful to grow in the shadows of death.

When my dear friend Rowen was diagnosed with cancer, my faith was tested yet again. To find out that another beloved friend was facing a serious cancer diagnosis at 46 was shocking! Rowen is not doing well. Her health is spiraling down and I will have to accept that another friend will soon die. During many months of her sickness, she lived twenty minutes away. I was helping her out with the necessary day-to-day tasks while undergoing my own natural cancer treatment protocol. Then she moved three hours away so that she could have around the clock care, which became necessary during her decline. I kept asking myself why I was facing the loss of my dearest friends at such a young age, while I myself am journeying with a serious health diagnosis?

I deeply trust that we are given what we can handle. I believe that all our trials and tribulations are gifts that ask us to grow. We can either step up to face the challenge and see the beauty in the twisted hero or heroine's path or we can contract in fear. My Kundalini yoga teacher, Jai Dev Singh Khalsa, says that if we are not doing our inner work then challenging circumstances, such as car accidents, sickness, and other incidents, will occur to stretch us. When yet another terribly hard circumstance occurs, it is a direct call to action, and to see each painful situation as an opportunity to transform. In order to cope with the arduous aspects of what life can bring, I chose to accept these painful situations as gifts that would help me grow.

Receiving a cancer diagnosis is tremendously challenging. As I've chosen to share my healing journey publicly through my Cancer Warrioress blog and Facebook page, I receive messages frequently from readers sharing how brave and inspirational they find me. My purpose in sharing my vulnerability is not to gain praise but to show how many choices there are in a path to healing. I know how extremely overwhelming it can be, when given a diagnosis, to make an authentic decision about treatments and a path of healing. The fear and projection from others is paralyzing, not to mention the grim message from standard doctors, suggesting that you will most likely die soon if you begin treatment right away. I think anyone who is journeying with cancer is extremely brave regardless of how they choose to treat themselves.

I chose to openly share my journey of witnessing my closest friend of nineteen years go through allopathic treatment, as it made such a dramatic impact on me. A new awareness began to form through this process of witnessing Deb and Rowen's different journeys around cancer. I began to develop compassion for those facing the very kind of decisions they both faced. In my situation, I not only had the benefit of my direct experiences of care giving for Deb, but I also have a natural stubbornness and a headstrong aspect to my personality and yet these decisions were still difficult for me. I knew it must be extra challenging for those who did not have my experience and were not also as naturally tenacious as I was.

With compassion, I speak to share, to inspire, and to create waves of knowledge so that others may know there are many options for healing. I am choosing my path because it is the right one for me. Someone else could take the same route, but unless they believed in it, it simply may not work. Choosing an allopathic path would not have cured me, as I do not believe in chemotherapy. We all have the right to choose the correct decision for ourselves. One decision is not better than another. This way of empowered choice is indeed the warrior's path, the hero's journey, and, in my case, the fast track for growth.

I stumbled upon Kundalini Yoga a few months before Deb was diagnosed with Leukemia. I was attending classes at my local yoga studio and was curious about the class where people were wearing white and chanting loudly. They also looked ecstatically blissful afterward. They had a certain glow about them, which intrigued me. I decided to try a class one day and immediately understood the power of this practice. Holding postures for long periods of time while deeply breathing and chanting was a bit mystifying, at first. But the sense of peace that resulted from this manner of challenge was renewing. I have felt regularly drawn to the spiritual side of life. Kundalini yoga, its beautiful music and mantras accompanying a class are deeply healing. I was fortunate to have found this way right before Deb was diagnosed. Her life was dangling by a thread and she was my closest friend. Kundalini yoga helped me face her illness.

In 1967, Yogi Bhajan brought Kundalini yoga to the US from India. It is a form of yoga that includes the chanting of mantras and songs to raise one's consciousness beyond the chatter of the mind. There are specific yogic exercises with each posture having a purpose. There are exercises for developing intuition, for clearing away energies of past partners, for strengthening willpower. It is a powerful way to harness one's strength.

I am grateful to have found such a vehicle for accessing my own inner voice at such a painful time in my life. On one hand, I was exhausted by caring for my friend, while I was simultaneously terrified of losing her. On the other hand, I was filled with such love and faith while experiencing this wonderful new practice. It was nourishing my spirit and allowing myself to see that there was actually a strange rhythm and reason to the pain that my dear friend was experiencing. I could see those reasons even through the grief I felt about possibly losing her. The songs, and the sense of release that I experienced after Kundalini yoga classes were immeasurably powerful.

The Kundalini yoga practice community that embraced me was a welcome gift during the stark reality that Deb might not survive beyond her 46th year. It allowed me to see that with hardship comes great beauty. Why else would I be given such a gift alongside such tragedy? The contrasts between these realities gave me faith that everything in life is divine. I understand now that even the hardest situations have benefits to offer to those that choose to see those benefits.

Recently, I was blessed to attend Sat Nam Festival, a five-day Kundalini Yoga and music festival held in Joshua Tree, California every April. I had attended the previous year and knew it would be a perfect retreat to restore my spiritual reserves, which I would need to draw from to get through the challenging parts of the journey still to come. During the festival, I was rejuvenated while hearing the top musicians in the Kundalini community and I was able to attend yoga classes with my favorite teachers. Just being surrounded by the beauty and power of the desert landscape was enough to propel me into new levels of grace-filled awareness.

I had a phenomenal insight related to the journey with cancer while listening to Snatam Kaur, originally one of the most famous Kundalini Yoga singers who were schooled by Yogi Bhajan himself. There is a beautiful term for the 'essence of all sound' in Kundalini Yoga, which is the word 'Naad'. Naad is also the vibrational harmony through which the infinite can be experienced. While swimming in the beautiful rhapsody of the Naad, a rush of awareness flooded over me. What if cancer was my ultimate teacher for growth? What if cancer was a gift to help bring me to my next stage of evolution? Maybe cancer is really a force of love and faith that has come my way to teach me the greatest lesson possible. I can either choose to dwell in the possibility of fear or the reality of love.

A cancer diagnosis can bring an immediate fear, as it did for me, as the medical establishment, society, family, and friends are all too willing to respond or react in fear, as well. The key to navigating this territory is recognizing that love dwells on the other side of fear and most importantly, so does faith. I found that the awareness I needed while traversing these events is to allow the beauty of love to stream not only into myself but also to others in my life.

Love is a healing force and there is an endless supply of it. If we truly capture the essence of love it can transcend all limitations and suffering. It taught me that there is a purpose for the pain that I was experiencing on so many different levels. Having allowed cancer to be my teacher, I know that I am so much more than my body and through that clear knowing, I know within myself that we all are infinite beings filled with such beauty and light. Allowing that beauty to fill our lives can be the force that heals all illnesses.

I have been willing to go against the grain in many situations in my life. Even when friends rally around something that is popular in mainstream media, I have chosen to follow my own path. My choice to heal my cancer naturally was no exception to the consistent way I have been living my life. I was able to make this unconventional choice by consistently monitoring my breast cancer with a highly refined test called the 'Greece' or RGCC test. This test measures the circulating tumor cell count in the bloodstream. It is not offered in the USA, which means the blood sample must be sent to Greece. Every three months I do the test to chart my progress.

The first time I did the test was November 2016 and my tumor cell count was at 8.2. This count showed a high amount of circulating tumor cells in my bloodstream. With a Stage three Breast Cancer diagnosis, I was not that surprised that my tumor cell count was as high as it was. The fact that the numbers were elevated was another reminder that I had a serious diagnosis, which was disheartening. The second time I took the test was in April, 2017. Those results showed my cell count dropped from 8.2 to 6.5, which was almost a two-point drop! The average drop for the protocol that I follow is one point every three months. Through my focused application of strict diet and natural protocol, I was showing nearly double the healing.

Oncologists in the USA cannot give results like this because the standard cancer care does not include the measurement of tumor cell counts. Although this method of measuring cancer is not yet accepted in mainstream American medicine, it is accepted and used successfully in other countries. It offers a way to monitor tumor cells rather than just using the traditional protocol.

What I have come to understand through my research around the RGCC test was that the cancer tumor cells that remain after chemotherapy and radiation wait in the bloodstream and can emerge even stronger and more resistant to chemotherapy in the future. Unfortunately, what many chemotherapy patients experience is that cancer cells return years later in a new organ or place in their body. With the support of the RGCC test, instead of focusing on killing and removing the tumor, I am working on reducing the tumor cells in my bloodstream. In this way, I am directly addressing the cause in this work with cancer.

My protocol is successful, yet the tumor over my breast remains. The view of my physicians is that a tumor of this size is too large to remove it with a lumpectomy. Their view suggested that it was better for me to elect chemotherapy to possibly shrink the tumor so that a lumpectomy could be performed. That leaves me with the general opinion of the allopathic community that I should have my entire breast removed with a mastectomy. If I do choose a mastectomy, it would be a choice to embrace the Amazon women warrior archetype, who remove a breast in order to use a bow and arrow more effectively.

Grandma Rita was the one grandparent, who was still alive when I was growing up. She was a Christian Scientist, and she lived in a mountain town in New Hampshire. Grandma Rita installed a sense of faith in the way she lived her life and through her spiritual outlook. As my parents held a scientifically based belief system, the only time I would go to Sunday school was with Grandma Rita when she visited us in California. She believed in the power of positive thought and I remember her often saying 'God is love'. As a child that made no sense to me, but when I grew older I was able to grasp the meaning of it. She carried a strong faith in her own ability to heal herself and those that she loved.

My dear Grandmother died at the age of 81 in 1990. Weeks before her death, in order to see her one more time, I drove across country from California to Massachusetts. We spent precious moments together, which I now regard was a commemoration of her life. We talked, I rubbed her feet and enjoyed our last moments together. I did not know that she would die a few days after I left, making that special time spent together even more of an honor and privilege. I realize twenty-seven years after her death that I draw upon the strength and deep faith that she carried for my own trials and tribulations in life. I will never forget the positive impact my Grandma Rita had upon my life.

The most difficult times of my cancer journey through natural healing are when there is a massive detoxification happening. Dead cancer cells cycle through my liver and I can feel quite terrible. Max Gerson, creator of a natural approach to curing cancer called the Gerson Method, calls these die-offs 'healing responses.' During these die-offs, I experience some or all of these symptoms: exhaustion, body aches, headache, fever, nausea, mood swings and so much more. I know these responses are temporary, but that does not make them easy to endure.

There are ways to make the detoxification cycle a bit easier, like sweating in an infrared sauna, coffee enemas, herbs and other routines, but healing responses are definitely the hardest part of my healing journey. Usually, once I get through the cell die-off detoxification symptoms, I feel great since my immune system is being strengthened.

When I'm feeling terrible physically, I have found that emotions such as depression, sadness, frustration, and anger need to be released in order to feel free in my body and mind. I believe that processing them is necessary for healing.

Sometimes my body hurts so much, I just feel like crawling into a hole and disappearing. In times like this, rest is necessary to allow the body to have its healing cycle. In these moments, my faith can certainly be pushed to its limits, and I wonder why I am struggling with a life threatening diagnosis at such a young age.

Thankfully I have the wise words of guidance from teachers and friends I look up to. They remind me to ask for help, to pray, to remember the source of who I am and where my center is. They whisper in my ear that I'm a spiritual being having a human experience. I know that our bodies are limited, but that our souls are from vast, uncharted territories that know no bounds or limits. I remind myself that even if I were to die from breast cancer, my spirit would be alive. In the big picture, I am just a tiny speck in an amazingly grand design.

In the darkest of moments, faith comes in and wraps me in her tender arms. Ultimately, I know I'm not alone. I am being accompanied throughout this treacherous path. Friends and family cannot walk with me, but they can hold beautiful space, protecting and supporting me.

Sometimes in the early hours of the night, around four or five a.m. I find myself wide awake. It is during these moments where I receive powerful messages, which help fuel this treacherous journey. I find that any unprocessed event, unsettled emotions, doubt or fear cascade through my mind, like waves on the ocean. It is then that I am asked to face my most challenging shadows. The quiet of the night is where the truth arises to bring light to the darkness.

One of the teachings that has stuck with me is to remember to ask my spirit guides, healthy ancestors, God, Goddess, or Great Spirit to give me sustenance when going through a challenging time. The early morning hours is the time for my strongest prayers. I ask for guidance and clarity to guide me through the rough times. I usually receive the answers I am looking for and gradually feel the layers of stress and tension melt away.

Faith moves the mountains otherwise stones are heavier for men. What is the power of the man, what his the real power of the person? Faith. What is the inner nature of the person? Faith. What is the essence of all knowledge? Faith. What is the greatest blessing of God? Faith. What is earned of everything? Faith. If you cannot have faith in self and you cannot give faith to others, you have not yet moved one step in life. - Yogi Bhajan, Los Angeles, May 31, 1976.

Including myself in this vision for a new way of healing, we are meant to grow, change, and rise to meet all adversity. Life is not stagnant and never will be. Faith is the flag I have chosen to carry through the toughest of times. Allowing myself to surrender in its arms, I am indeed held, no matter what the outcome will be. In fact, I'm grateful for the lessons of cancer, as I would not have had the opportunity for such immense growth. Illness has allowed me to embrace my own vulnerability. I now understand how fragile and precious life is and cherish every moment. Without the deaths of my beloved friends and my own cancer diagnosis, I would not have understood the great power of faith. Ultimately this belief evokes grace. I sail in the arms of grace to return to full health once again, trusting that I am already healed.

Sweet Surviving, Spirited Thriving
by Pamela A. Smith, SS.C.M., Ph.D.

When I attended the 50th reunion of my high school class with roughly 140 of 330 classmates, I found that only a few had not quite gotten over the Age of Aquarius. One of them, our ace visual artist, still wore the long hair and the peasant style dress we associate with the late 1960's. Another friend with whom I had a charmed reunion, now lived with his wife in Maine, had published some scathing social criticism and fine poetry, and apparently lived with a degree of voluntary poverty. Among us were physicians, dentists, grocers, cosmetologists, lawyers, mechanics, attorneys, engineers, owners of businesses, cabinet makers, teachers, musicians, and retired government workers; one, who offered the invocation, was a minister. Most of us had become part of the middle class, and the Establishment.

We had lost 40 classmates to Vietnam, auto accidents, kidney disease, leukemia, heart disease, and a variety of undisclosed causes. Despite that, it seemed that everyone present had weathered family problems, disillusionments, yet formed lasting relationships, many with their original spouses, and also settled into contentment.

My own journey differed considerably from the rest. True, I had washed pots and sold Avon, and had then gone on to teach every level from eighth grade through graduate school, to hold a variety of administrative positions, to serve as president of several boards, and to write articles, poems, and books. But I was the only nun in the room, and, as I learned well into the evening gala, I was the last surviving Type 1 diabetic among my classmates. There had been two others that I had known of, both diagnosed some years before I was. Both had died in 2011.

Events like class reunions seem to create an onslaught of nostalgia, regret, grief, gratitude, and wonder. As I approach another 50th anniversary, that of the diagnosis of the disease that has charted my life, I find myself looking back at that life's turns and twists. I notice that some experiences of what I could have accomplished still sting, but find blessings and little triumphs are cause for celebration. A mix of grit and grace is a central part of my story of illness.

At onset, it was clear that diabetes mellitus, Type 1, then called juvenile diabetes, was not easy to grasp or face. To this day, it is not easy to live with or through.

Sometime in October 1969 I had a strange rash. I went to the general practitioner, an osteopath, whom I saw regularly for recurrent sinus infections, received an antibiotic, and the rash disappeared. I was teaching in a rough and tumble public school, had started graduate studies with an 80-mile commute every Tuesday night and Saturday morning. I was dating sporadically in the aftermath of an engagement I had broken, writing poetry, and making pilgrimages to the Philadelphia Museum of Art. Fatigue had become a way of life.

Over the Thanksgiving break I visited my mother and family in Berwick, PA, and was bystander to an event called the annual Race for Diamonds, a mini-marathon. Somehow the faces in the crowd across the street looked blurred. As I drove back to the Philadelphia area that Sunday, I noticed that I wasn't seeing the usually very discernible signs on the PA Turnpike very clearly. Then, as the week progressed, I had trouble focusing on students in the back of the room, and shifting from close-up printed page to distance vision. I suspected that I needed new glasses. I was ravenously hungry, no matter what I ate, and very thirsty. As I dressed for work one morning, I noticed that my skirt seemed a bit loose. I had unaccountably lost ten pounds.

Every day my second period was free. My department chairperson walked into the English center and found me dozing Friday morning. He asked how I was feeling, since he had noticed I didn't look quite right. Then he happened to mention that a friend's teen-age son had just been diagnosed with diabetes after having been mistakenly treated for viruses or flu for weeks and wound up in the hospital. I went to the school library, picked up a medical reference book, and found that I could make check marks by the list of symptoms of diabetes. I called the doctor, went to his office immediately after school, uttered an expletive when he told me his conclusions from a hastily done urine test. By early evening

I was a patient at Delaware Valley Hospital getting my first doses of insulin, and having my first experience of insulin shock as the injected units jolted my whole system.

Over an eight-day period I learned to give myself shots and urine tests to see whether I was spilling sugar, bought a few days of iron to remedy anemia, and was x-rayed to be sure that I didn't have pancreatic cancer. My landlady brought changes of pajamas plus my portable typewriter and notes and books. I received permission, despite hospital roommates who might have been understandably dismayed, to type my final papers for my graduate English classes. Then I called the department chair and received an extension for taking exams, as well as hosting a handful of students from my sophomore honors English class when they decided to come for a visit.

I read voraciously, including a number of books about diabetes and its treatment. Much of what I read may have been designed to terrify patients into compliance, something I was naturally inclined to anyway. I learned about the discovery of insulin, the difference between juvenile and older adults with this illness, how to calculate meal exchanges and factor in exercise. I also read about how to prepare the diabetic for the likelihood of a shortened life, or a life with significant disability; an 80 percent chance of damage to the retinas after 20 years, a 40 percent chance of heart disease, amputation, dialysis, and neuropathy the likely future of a long-term diabetic. On the other hand, it might help to try hard, the books suggested, though the medical evidence was still out on whether maintaining near normal blood sugars could stave off these complications.

On the outside, I was just busy getting back to business as usual, to the illusory sense that it was possible. A few months down the road, when I confessed to my physician that I was "kind of depressed," he responded that it was about time. I had adapted, he said, almost too well. In other words, I was doing what I had to do to stay alive and functional, but I was pretending that it didn't particularly faze me.

Keeping active in the hospital helped me with my depression. I had cried in the middle of the week there, feeling vulnerable and abandoned in the middle of one very bad night. The next day I asked if I could volunteer to do something until I was released, and I began by delivering mail to patients' rooms. Plus, I wrote my papers, finished my courses, and gave my students their end of quarter reports and exams, all the while acting as though not much had changed. Except that I now had a life-threatening disease; demanding measured amounts of insulin and food, urine tests done with test tubes and tablets in the bathroom at home every day, regular blood tests in a hospital laboratory, and quarterly, if not more frequent, visits to a well-trained general practitioner. or endocrinologist. And, because of the risk of hypoglycemia, and the fact that I was starting to fit the profile of a "brittle" diabetic, I had to be sure I had a reachable supply of candy, juice, and snacks that could raise my blood sugar at all times. I had to tell my colleagues and students that I was diabetic so that they would know what to do in case of an emergency.

One of the consequences of learning that my life might be considerably shorter than average or my ability to function might be severely curtailed was a redirection of my plans. For some time I had known that teaching, writing, and human service were my passions. I wasn't so sure that a public high school with racial tensions, and an undercurrent of drug abuse and vandalism was the place for me now. I also wasn't sure in whom or what to invest my trust and commitments. I wanted to help people think, have regard for one another, and live together harmoniously. I had a yearning for transcendence but was not sure what I believed, beyond being gripped by William Blake's yen "To see a world in a grain of sand/ And a heaven in a wild flower,/Hold infinity in the palm of your hand/And eternity in an hour." I decided that I should probably become a college professor and completed the application for a teaching assistantship while still in the hospital. But there were spiritual matters which eventually would become an important part of my life.

From the time I was seven years old, I knew that I had an attraction to miracle and mystery. It ranged from an episode on "Rin-Tin-Tin" to the Bible and stories about saints I heard in Catholic grade school. On one episode of the aforementioned TV program, young Rusty, always in the company of his beloved

German shepherd Rinny and aware of Apache legendry, was caught in a buffalo stampede. At the critical moment, the stampede suddenly stopped when a white buffalo appeared. A Native American elder had told Rusty of white buffalos and how they mystically came to favored persons. Rusty's life was saved, and no one else had seen the vision or could explain the sudden paralysis of the herd. I wanted nothing more than to see a white buffalo.

Around the same time, I also decided that I wanted to cross the Grand Central Parkway service road to attend early morning Mass because there was something mystical about that too. It was held in Latin, and people buried their heads in their hands after Communion. Pigeons and doves frequented our Queens, New York city neighborhood, and I almost always met some of them along the way to or from St. Nick's. I felt sure that one of them would be the Holy Ghost, and hoped that I would recognize that Spirit, who was also God.

My spiritual path did not stay on a particular route to sanctity, however. As a child and a youth I attended my church every Sunday. My father's death when I was fourteen years old, and a mounting sense of national tragedy from the Cuban missile crisis to a series of assassinations, to a war that triggered social upheaval catapulted my whole generation into tense questioning. As I moved into young adulthood, I started introducing African and African American literature into my students' course of studies. I also tried, off hours, to determine if I were Unitarian, Protestant, or agnostic, all while holding on to an appreciation of Catholicism with a small "c."

When I was saddled with a disease that many expected would disable me by the time I was in my forties, I was in the agnostic phase, wanting to do something to make the world a better and more peaceful place, but uncertain where to focus. Around that time while I was in graduate school, I met a Mennonite conscientious objector, two Baptists who were knowledgeable about racial justice, peacemaking, and advancing the status of women. I also met Catholic sisters who studied, taught, were engaged in creative projects, and were heavily invested in the *aggiornamento,* the updating that Pope John XXIII and Vatican II, about which I understood precious little.

When I moved into a Puerto Rican neighborhood in my third year of living with a serious illness, I found an apartment a half block from Holy Infancy Church, *Santa Infancia*, surrounded by backstreets, the parish's used clothing store, and restaurants like El Caribe where one could eat beans and rice and a little meat for a pittance. I was in a Ph.D. program in English with a graduate teaching assistantship at Lehigh University living in space that cost eleven dollars a week to rent. However, I had to sell my car and use a bicycle to be able to afford what were then incredibly inexpensive syringes and insulin siphoned from beef and pork pancreases. I walked a lot too. In between studies and writing papers and teaching, I began pondering the first twenty psalms, read them in English and Spanish, and suddenly understood what it meant to encounter the Living Word. The person of Jesus inexplicably came to life, almost in the air, and I began to associate resurrection with people I encountered in my little barrio, the drug addicts, the alcoholics, the Puerto Ricans tinkering with their cars, the children spilling out of tumble-down houses. I headed back to church, meditated without knowing quite how, and determined that some dramatic counter-cultural move was demanded by my new discipleship.

I didn't think that diabetes had much to do with it, but it clearly inspired me to do what I could when it was possible. There was a sense of urgency in our country, but there was also an exaggerated sense of urgency in me. Always just below the surface I felt, and, though I would never admit it, feared the pulse of hypo-sugared blood and already experienced the daze of overdose and sugar gone way too low. I didn't know how much time there might be to do anything constructive, creative, humanitarian, or meaningful. At that time, people who lived in Monasteries, Buddhist or Christian, seemed to be engaged in more profound work. We had seen them in action as Vietnam unfolded, the ones who had burned themselves out serving or who had literally burned themselves to death in order to protest bombing, strafing, and napalm.

It has been forty five years since I entered the community of the Sisters of Saints Cyril and Methodius, a group founded in 1909 in Pennsylvania by Slovak immigrants. The community's mission, in contemporary terms, can be summed up in evangelization, education, elder care, and ecumenism. The patron saints, the ninth century apostles to the Slavic peoples, were Greek brothers who created the Cyrillic alphabet, translated the gospels into Old Slavonic, devised a sacred liturgy in that same language, and cultivated catechists and clergy among people who were considered peasants. They were 1100 years ahead of their times because they promoted widespread literacy, focused on making Scripture accessible to many, created a Mass in the vernacular, honored the traditions and customs of the people as they Christianized them. They also focused on training and mentoring leaders for their native country. This is what Catholicism's Vatican II concluded in 1965 and had emphasized as essential to mission.

Of the two brothers, Methodius was the one who had been a civic official in Byzantium before he became a priest, missionary, and bishop. He was a trained and accomplished administrator. Cyril was called the philosopher, who taught in the emperor's court, enjoyed scholarship, and became a monk as well as the translator. While I have held a number of administrative positions, I have always found a soul brother in Cyril across the years. If I had to sum up my life project it would be translating the gospel to my contemporaries. Sometimes they have been youths, sometimes adults, sometimes readers, sometimes attendees at crowded or very small events, as well as people who never went to church, and people who regularly attended mass.

Within the past two months I have received an award and have been told I would be getting a couple of new writing contracts. I have reviewed budget proposals with campus ministers, youth and young adult ministers, a school superintendent, and faith formation directors. I have offered reflections on African saints at a Black Heritage Month day of prayer and conducted a short retreat at an eco-spiritual center hosting a group of sisters from Canada, Australia, Kenya, and the U.S.

I have also met two homeless men with whom I exchanged stories and prayed, men whom I met because I passed them on crowded streets and in close quarters, and turned back to approach them. One, who asked why I stopped and wept when I told him I saw Jesus in his eyes. Of these events, it is obvious that all of them have mission and ministry about them. But the last ones, the street encounters, may have been the most important and most valuable to me, to Terry and Sam, and to all three of us.

Being diabetic so long may have nothing to do with that evaluation. But I have a feeling that a certain sympathy with the invisible man or woman or child comes more easily if one has had to wake up every day to one's own fragility and temporality. There's a brokenness that comes of having a bothersome chronic disease, and the best thing to do with that brokenness is to perceive and empathize with someone else's brokenness. In some ways, that's the summary of my spirituality. The Spirit of God is everywhere and in everyone.

My religious community does not come from the tradition inspired by St. Francis of Assisi, but that patron saint of ecology has touched my life. He desired simplicity and felt wed to what he called *Lady Poverty*. I am working on that, but I have to admit that my convent life has not lacked for comforts. I live, after all, in a multi-racial middle-class neighborhood near Savannah and Hilton Head. I've enjoyed advantages in terms of conferences and retreats and opportunities to live and work in four states in the U.S. and also, twice, to see Rome. So the desire for simplicity and simplifying are there, but not altogether realized. If my community or I were radically poor, I would have died for lack of medical equipment and medical care. Where the spirit of Francis has most surely touched me, though, has been in my interest in environmental ethics and eco-spirituality, that I taught and wrote about. It has also been part of my volunteering at the St. Francis Center at St. Helena Island, South Carolina, an outreach center particularly serving the poor among the island Gullah population, and Spanish-speaking migrant workers who come to plant and pick tomatoes.

My love for the Old and New Testaments has been a source of inspiration, adaptation, and creative writing for me, as well as a source for many workshops and days of recollection. From poring over psalms in Bethlehem, Pennsylvania, decades ago to the present day, I continue to find in the words of the Bible, the human experience of agony and ecstasy, and genuine encounters with truth and the God of life. Scripture, and the regular rhythms of personal and community prayer and public worship, give me stability and strength for the day and for the years ahead. I think very rarely of eternal life, which might seem a surprising admission from a fervent Christian, but it seems that my attunement to the present has grown sharper with my growth in faith. Paradoxically, perhaps, the here and now has become more riveting in the aftermath of setbacks, near-misses that could have been deadly, and blessed recovery. I'm also fascinated with the realm of religious experience and thus have been interested in Zen, Islam, Judaism, and varieties of Christian belief. There is a healing togetherness which I have found in official dialogues and in simple trading of ideas and questions, one on one. Encountering more deeply the souls of others, and touching both their convictions and their uncertainties has had the effect of freeing me to be, as Robert Frost termed it, "one acquainted with the night" and to be quite at peace with the daily round.

My years as a diabetic have required routines of shots, stints on insulin pumps and glucose sensors, blood tests, and corrections for the inevitable trial-and-error of this disease. Medical advances have improved diabetes care tremendously, starting with the development of DNA recombinant human insulin, and the stress of self-management. Flexibility in meal contents and meal times has made it easier to change schedules and time zones. Yet, the life of a diabetic is not easy, but is always somehow edgy. Being a brittle diabetic is being different. No matter how independent one presumes or prefers to be, interdependence and dependence are key. The interdependence is on medical procedures, family, friends, colleagues and on at least four occasions, emergency rooms. The dependence is on those who are caregivers when we can't help ourselves. And it's also dependence on the goodness of creation and of God, even while the ability to understand how both operate eludes us in so many ways.

We all know that we are mortal. Some think about it more than once in a lifetime. For me, the fact that I could die any day as a result of one false move or one small error has at times been chilling. Generally, though, it is a fact of life with which I have attained as more than a truce. If I die suddenly, it will be no one's fault. If I live to be 122 for, say, the 100th anniversary of my diabetes, it will be no one's real credit. It will be the vagaries of a world as St. Thomas Aquinas long ago declared, chance as part of God's providential design.

Meanwhile, I have learned to be busy and, as I get very close to turning 70, to be convinced that sometimes one can do more by doing a little less. I have also learned to revel in the ordinary. Author Kathleen Norris has praised what she terms "the quotidian mysteries," the mysteries of the everyday. While I continue to minister actively, I find myself more and more appreciating the beauty and significance of sunrise over Port Royal Sound, the snuffing of our rescue dog named Angel, the swoop of herons and pelicans and wood storks and the splay of cormorant wings, the fronds of the dwarf palmetto, and the patter of neighbors who don't necessarily speak my native language. Realizing that I can see, taste, smell, feel, hear, walk, sing, and think renders me grateful.

Years ago, our convent libraries all participated in a book club which sent a book by Brother David Steindl-Rast one particular month. It was entitled *Gratefulness: The Heart of Prayer*. I have never forgotten the title because gratitude now seems to be the central theme of my life. I am no longer the child who longs for white buffaloes or apparitions of the Holy Spirit. Instead, I find myself actively content to live, to keep working at it, and to enjoy it to the hilt. That seems holy and altruistic enough. And it seems to be a way of meeting, bearing, and being a Body of Christ in a tremulous world.

Performance Art, Illness, and My Desert Prayer
by Neil Ellis Orts

A brother said to Abba Anthony, "Pray for me." The old man said to him, "I will have no mercy upon you, nor will God have any, if you yourself do not make an effort and if you do not pray to God."

I first became aware of the Desert Fathers and Mothers sometime in the late 1980s, when I was going through a Thomas Merton phase in my spiritual reading. I picked up his *The Wisdom of the Desert* and was intrigued by the short sayings and stories I found therein. I expanded my reading to the many books by Benedicta Ward, Helen Waddell, and others. Roberta Bondi's first book on them, *To Love as God Loves*, has been one of the few books in my library that I have read front to back multiple times. I found these desert dwellers puzzling, funny, and profound. They are my spiritual heroes that accompanied me when I most needed them.

One gave me a prayer to anchor me through a health scare. February 4, 2013, I went to my cardiologist's office to get the results of a CT scan on my heart. Dr. Andrew Civitello had ordered the CT because I'd said I "felt something," but also that I didn't think it was my heart. "If I had to guess," I'd said, "I'd say it was a gastrointestinal thing."

He sat down and told me that my heart looked fine, nothing new to see there. However, when they took the pictures of my heart, they caught a portion of my pancreas but only a portion. Still, it looked like there was something there that shouldn't be. With a tone that seemed to be testing my knowledge of his comments, he added, "We think you should have that looked at." And I agreed. I saw in his face that he understood that I had, and that he had efficiently communicated the gravity of the moment. He then said, "I've already contacted Dr. Kneitz and he's working on a referral for you."

Despite the news I'd just received, I couldn't help but smile, thankful for my primary care physician, Dr. Joel Kneitz, and my cardiologist. My doctors were already sharing information about me, setting things in motion to help me before I knew I needed the help.

My experience with cancer was not minimal. When I attended seminary, I did a summer of Clinical Pastoral Education on a cancer floor in a hospital. My father had survived two cancers, colon and prostate, before dying suddenly after several years, cancer free. My mother died of lymphoma. Other cancers were in the family history and I had remarked on occasion that we each chose our own form of the disease. Had I chosen pancreatic cancer?

I called the Reverend Lisa Hunt, the rector at the church I was attending. I had told her that I was having the heart CT done and she'd asked me to call her when I found out the results. She has a particular gift for being pastoral while also being very direct. Her first words upon hearing my news were, "Oh Neil, that's not good." "I know!" I replied into my cell phone. I smiled again, glad that I didn't have to explain it. And what else could she say to the news but, "You'll be in my prayers."

This wasn't my first brush with mortality. This mass was found, after all, by my cardiologist, who I see regularly because, in 2006, I had a completely clogged artery on my heart. But that clogged artery business had been very different. Yes, it had lots of follow up and self-monitoring, but the symptoms, diagnosis, and solution to the problem all occurred within four days. In fact, the clogged artery was discovered and opened via a stint all in one morning. I didn't have time for mystery in that case. I didn't have time to worry.

Nothing happens in a vacuum because the performance installation I was creating at the time was more than relevant. Ironically, it was called Shadow Place, and created as a meditation on light and shadow. It had six performers, two carrying small but very bright lights and four who carried two translucent fabric screens. The screens moved and were always separating the two light-carriers. The lights created shadows and partial glimpses through the screens. Even more, the site for the installation was a storefront venue with glass on three sides, on a busy street in

Houston. I scheduled the installation for evenings as the sun was setting so that natural light decreased and the lights from passing traffic added random shadows to the ones created by the performers. It was designed, really, to be watched outside the venue by walking passersby as they went to and from the nearby restaurants. It would run three Sunday evenings during the season of lent.

Of course, the fact that I was in the midst of creating a performance installation called Shadow Place while dealing with a mass on my pancreas was not lost on me. A meditation on darkness and light? I suddenly felt much more connected to my own work.

On February 11, my cast had our second rehearsal and I told my collaborators about this medical kink in my plans. I had considered canceling Shadow Place, and focus on the health issues, rather than risk being incapacitated by chemotherapy in the middle of rehearsals or performances. But, I decided not to stop the performance, but to keep going.

A recurring question for artists, from others and to ourselves, is, "Where do ideas come from?" Where did an idea for shadow and light play with fabric and passing traffic come from? What made me decide to do a meditative performance installation with the darkness falling as it progressed? Shadow Place? It seems too much of a coincidence to have this all come up at a time I had a pancreatic mass. As a Christian, I believe my whole body is part of my identity. Incarnational theology, it seems to me, might suggest that our whole being, physical as well as mental or spiritual, is the site of contemplation.

Being trained in the theater, with some dance experience, and then making performance art---all bodily art forms---coupled with my theological education, I tend to think about things like stage presence. This intangible projection to the back row of the theater, must surely have something to do with spirit. Or I think about muscle memory, how meat and bone hold past practices and events. I have no problem entertaining the notion that there is some overlap between what we call the subconscious with our physical body, that our flesh can be involved in the act of thinking.

Was my pancreas informing my creative process? I'm willing to entertain the notion.

I also felt my whole physical self "thinking" in my dreams. One dream was something I didn't participate in, I only watched it. It had the feel of a 1970s made-for-TV movie, with dramatic close-ups and the styles were from that period. The setting was the rooftop of a tall, urban building. A teenaged girl stood on the edge of the building, facing the roof, her back to the street. She was trying to decide what to do, whether to jump or not. She was barefoot and only had one foot on the ledge and just the ball of that foot. The toes of the other foot tapped the ledge as she considered her options. Below her, not on the ground, but somewhere somewhat precarious, too, was an adult man, unidentified, who tried to talk her out of jumping. I never saw her jump, neither did I see her step onto the roof to safety, just the close-ups of her feet, the one foot tapping the ledge in indecision.

The other dream took place in a church, one I used to attend. The pastor from that congregation was there and also another man, who was an amalgam of a couple of different parishioners. This third man was supposed to lie in a shallow, pretend coffin. It was shaped like an old wooden coffin, narrow at the head and feet, broad at the shoulders. I had moved it up towards the altar, but the pastor said it could be farther back in the congregation. I wasn't getting a clear idea of what that meant because it was as obviously intended to be a prop for a sermon illustration. While I tried to figure that out, a little girl, about five, blonde-haired, crawled into the coffin, played dead, and then giggled. At some point, I realized the coffin lid was hinged incorrectly. When viewing a body, the coffin is hinged so the head is to the left of the viewer. This was oriented with the head to the right.

That's all I recorded of the dreams, but they stayed with me, felt like more than my ordinary dreams. Two days later, I wondered if my body/subconscious was trying to tell me that this pancreas business was serious but not deadly. It was play acting at death, but was ultimately not anything more serious than a sermon illustration. I didn't know if I was grasping at straws or accurately interpreting my dreams, but it calmed my nerves to think of it this way. It gave me some comfort.

I've always put any art project, whatever the genre, as my priority. Now, I had this thing that was taking priority even over my creative endeavors. At the same time, it was impossible to ignore that it does not shift everyone's priorities. Most frustrating was not finding myself to be the doctors' priority. I admit, I did not help this.

I got my referral from Dr. Kneitz, but I couldn't get in to see the oncologist -- a title I didn't like thinking about -- for nearly two weeks, and even then it was only for a consultation. I didn't understand why I wasn't immediately given an appointment for a biopsy, and it created more worries for me.

There's nothing to worry about. If there was, I'd already be in surgery, but since I'm not in surgery, there's nothing to worry about!

There's nothing to be done, so why rush? I'm doomed, so they may as well prioritize people they can actually help.

Intellectually, I knew there was more to it than either of those extremes could cover, and yet the emotions were in charge here, not the intellect. I kept enough wits about me to find most of my anxious fantasies darkly amusing. Even so, I must have been more upset than I wanted to admit. What else would explain my carelessness with my first oncologist appointment?

February 15, 2013, I was on a bus, on my way to meet the oncologist and my phone rang. It was his office. "You had an appointment for 9:40 and we're wondering what happened." "I thought it was 10:40," I answered. "No sir." I was 20 minutes late. After some failed negotiations, I was told I would be too late to be worked into that day's schedule. I had to reschedule for February 21.

This was clearly my fault. I looked again at my calendar---the same place I'd double checked the address!---and saw that I had, indeed, written down 9:40. Why did I think it was 10:40? Whatever self-sabotaging tendencies I have were in overdrive that day. To say I spent some time beating myself up over this would be an understatement.

I made arrangements at work for another absence and the next week I took extra special care to catch an early bus and get to the oncologist. He mainly asked questions about what I was experiencing. Then he asked me if I'd seen the CT scan that showed the mass. I hadn't, so he led me to another room and pulled my scan up on a computer screen.

A CT scan is basically taking multiple x-rays of an area, very slim slices at a time, each image after another slice through the body. He pointed to the portion of my pancreas caught in this scan and then he pointed out when the mass appeared in the succeeding images. As the pictures progressed, we watched the mass, what we could see of it, grow bigger and then smaller as the scan passed through it. I asked about the scale of the images we were watching. He said the pictures were close to actual size. The mass was about the size of a baseball.

"That seems like a fairly big mass," I said tentatively. As kindly as he could, he answered, "Yes, it is."

Abba Macarius was asked "How should one pray?" The old man said, "There is no need at all to make long discourses; it is enough to stretch out one's hand and say, 'Lord, as you will, and as you know, have mercy.' And if the conflict grows fiercer say: 'Lord, help.' He knows very well what we need and he shows us his mercy."

The Abbas and Ammas teach us much about prayer and speak often about death. They taught the importance of keeping death ever before us, as a way to maintain courage in the face of struggle. Prayer is to be practiced in all times, and is the means to combat all manner of spiritual and physical worries.

At the same time, anyone who is a religious person comes up against the problem of unanswered prayers. After all these years, including a seminary degree, and my brief time as a cancer floor chaplain, I admit I'm not always certain how to pray or what prayer even does. For this reason I sometimes describe myself as a prayer agnostic. I'm uncertain about the efficacy of prayer.

And yet, I believe in God and that belief tends toward a prayer component. My spiritual heroes talked incessantly about prayer. Having a mass on my pancreas seemed very worthy of prayer. But how does one pray about these things? I was reticent to pray for something---complete healing or the disappearance of the mass--- that I knew was unlikely. I wanted a practical prayer life in the face of this.

What's more, I don't hold to any illusions about being immune to awful things. Back in 2001, I recall hearing questions like "Where was God on 9/11?" I was infuriated by that question because behind it is the thought that God was somehow absent when this awful thing happened on U.S. soil. I believe that God is always where God is: With the oppressed, the suffering, the dying. If we fail to have crises of faith over a genocide in Rwanda, how dare we have a crisis of faith because a terrorist attack happened to us? I wasn't willing to go to the "why me?" question in my moment of potentially mortal illness. There is never any real answer to it anyway.

But the prayer of Macarius made sense to me. I could sincerely pray those words without expectations for unlikely miracles but still with hope for God to be present and active in this situation.

"Oh Lord, as you will and as you know, have mercy on me. Help me." This became my constant prayer, a mantra if you will. I even set it to music so I could sing and hum it as I took walks or did other activities of little concentration. I find it a couple of times in my journals, in the midst of everything else I recorded at the time.

My 50th birthday was coming up in October that year. I had started thinking about it, how I wanted to celebrate half a century. That now seemed questionable. As much as I reminded myself, several times a day, that we didn't know what the mass was, I couldn't help but wonder if I'd live until October. Ash Wednesday that year was February 13, two days before my missed oncologist appointment. Remember I was dust? Yes, I was on that.

I started thinking about who might be able to take my cat. I began thinking about who might want some of my books. I thought about some friends who had a little girl who was turning seven years old that year. I would be her first death. I reasoned I was a better candidate for that than, say, a grandparent, but how should I handle dying for her? My question wasn't "why me?" My question was, "If I'm dying, how do I do it?"

Serious illness is often met with words like "courageous," or "strong." These are qualities that are worth cultivating. We call them virtues. I found myself wondering what that looked like in my situation. My education and reading in performance theory, which has to do with all our roles in life, not just what happens on a stage, led me to questions like, "How does one perform courage? How shall I convey strength?" Which isn't to say courage and strength are simply poses we strike. They be learned, practiced, embodied qualities, authentic performances we give every day.

And I asked myself these questions because I think how we face personal issues such as a mass on a pancreas could be some kind of witness or even model to those around us. I think it's helpful to other people, regardless of religion, to see a way to react to life-threatening news that isn't simply falling apart.

But honestly, I can't say I was immediately on board with the strong and brave thing. I don't know that I ever really fell apart, but I definitely had a few days when I was preoccupied with ending my life. That was frightening and a little infuriating. But then we probably know that fear and anger are often sibling emotions, if not two sides of the same coin.

Mixing metaphors aside, I began to think that there was also a way to admit to being vulnerable and scared. To say anything else is, indeed, play-acting, performing in a less authentic sense of the word. As I like to say, denial is a defense mechanism, and we sometimes need defenses, but I also knew that it was not a place to stay. If I was to be strong and brave, there was a journey to make through admitting that I was weak, vulnerable, scared. And really, if the situation wasn't scary, what did I need courage for?

Oh Lord, as you will and as you know . . .

At the end of that first visit with the oncologist, I had blood work drawn. We set an appointment for a new, pancreas-centered CT for the next day, February 22. A biopsy was scheduled for February 28.

The first hopeful news came on February 26, two days before my biopsy. I received a phone call that told me that the blood work from the 21st showed no markers for pancreatic cancer. They stressed that it was not conclusive, that I still needed to have the biopsy, but they wanted to give me that much news.

The biopsy was a less amusing experience than a CT. They had to hook me up with all manner of wires to monitor my body functions as they did the procedure. The I.V. needle wouldn't go into my hand correctly and it took three different people to finally hit the vein. When they gave me an oxygen tube to put in my nose, I had a momentary feeling of panic. It's harder to distract myself with thoughts of time machines with an oxygen tube around my face. This was serious business.

The procedure wasn't awful, but it was uncomfortable. I felt the needle or tube or whatever it was enter my body and while I was unclear on the exact pathway into my anatomy, I felt like it was pressing against my diaphragm somehow. I found it difficult to take deep breaths without pain. "Mr. Orts, you're going to hear a some clicks." I guessed the clicks were the instrument inside me taking tiny bites off the mass.

After it was over, I asked if I could see what they took out of me. They held up a specimen jar, about the size used to collect urine samples. In it was a clear liquid and in the liquid floated tiny pink flecks.

Then the doctor doing the procedure said something remarkable. He said, "I don't think you have cancer." I was surprised that he would say that, as doctors are usually so careful not to jump to conclusions, particularly in our litigious society. Still, he performed biopsies all the time and so I guess he had an idea of what cancerous tissue looked like. I took what comfort I could from that. The results from the biopsy, they said, would take about a week.

More waiting.

O Lord, as you will and as you know . . .

Meanwhile, work continued on Shadow Place. I had a rehearsal scheduled for the day of my biopsy. I was supposed to go home directly from the hospital, but of course, I stopped by the venue to watch a bit of the rehearsal and give notes. I wasn't there for the whole rehearsal, so I felt I almost obeyed orders.

The first performance was scheduled for March 3. I was still enjoying that process, distracted as I was. The usual difficulties and frustrations of preparing a performance were present--- scheduling a cast of busy performers for rehearsals, communicating with the venue, figuring out publicity---but the work itself was pleasing me.

At this time, I was also beginning to present solo performance work with a new group in Houston called Continuum. They were having a series of monthly performance art evenings at a local venue, Avant Garden, and I'd presented a piece for the February show. The March show was coming up the Friday before the Shadow Place opening. Of course, I wanted to do something about my pancreas.

After considering and discarding a few ideas, I hit upon a piece I called Tell Me Where It Hurts. It was an interactive performance wherein I asked audience members who were patrons at Avant Garden, which is also a bar, to mark on my body in places where they had pains or scars, particularly things that no one could see. I dressed in a spandex body suit that covered me head to foot and that created me as a walking, talking blue silhouette. I handed people Sharpie pens to place an X on me, as well as a number between one and ten, one being low pain, ten being acute pain. I told the story of my pancreas---this was the day after my biopsy--- and placed a mark on my left side, where the needle went in, as I was still sore there. Then people made their marks. It felt like I was becoming a map of all the hidden pains and scars of the people in the bar that night. It felt like I was using my own health scare to facilitate other people's expression of health issues. It felt good, like a redemption activity for my own problems.

While I did perform in the opening of Shadow Place, I was able to simply sit and watch that first Sunday. I did my best to watch it with as calm a mind as I could. I was so pleased with the work. The moving fabric screens and the lights shining in the darkening space created great shadows throughout the room. The light from the passing traffic outside created a chaotic sense about where light came from. An artist can never be sure how something speaks to an audience but to me, it was all the symbolism of my current moment put on display. From health issues to that hour's conflict about prices, I had light in the darkness, often from unexpected places. Yes, I was so very pleased.

The next week, things happened quickly in roller coaster fashion. On March 4, 2013, the day after Shadow Place opened, I got a phone call from the oncologist's office. The samples they took did not show any sign of cancer. Obviously I was relieved. They said there was no need to see the oncologist again and instead I had an almost immediate appointment with a surgeon at Baylor College of Medicine. I met Dr. George Van Buren, II, on March 6.

In the two days between the biopsy news and meeting Dr. Van Buren, I felt so much relief. Surely I was in the clear with only the discomfort of a surgery to look forward to. I imagined that the surgery would only be some small incision through which they'd remove the cyst, laparoscopically, and then I would be fine. This only showed my great ignorance about what was going on.

Dr. Van Buren drew a picture of the pancreas, explained what this banana-shaped organ did, how it attached to the greater digestive system, and marked where my cyst was located. The good news was that my cyst was on the tail of the pancreas, the far end of the banana, away from where it connected to the rest of the digestive tract. This would make the cyst easier to remove and so the very best location for it. Removing cysts or tumors closer to the connecting end were much trickier operations although also successfully completed.

The bad news was that it was still a big operation. Cutting into the pancreas has its dangers. This would not be a laparoscopic procedure, but a more invasive surgery, with a hospital stay of four to seven days. They would have to monitor me these first days to make sure the incisions into the pancreas held, as leaking pancreatic juices would have dire circumstances. Then, after my hospital stay, I needed to prepare for two more weeks, minimum, out of work, but it ended up being three. I would be busy with a lot of healing.

Perhaps because I'd been so relieved that there was no sign of cancer, I wasn't quite prepared for all this very serious information. I understood that Dr. Van Buren has to tell his patients all the ways things can go wrong, and I knew almost all of them were unlikely. He is an experienced surgeon in a world class medical facility. He said he performed these surgeries on Tuesdays and Thursdays. I had every reason to think I'd just be another day in the office for him.

But three weeks, minimum, out of work? This was much more than just showing up, having a cyst scraped off an organ, and being on my way. I pulled out my calendar. I had two more Sundays for Shadow Place performances. I had a commitment to lead a performance workshop at Austin Community College the first week of April. I said the earliest I could do the operation and fulfill current commitments was April 9. Dr. Van Buren said that was fine, that there was no immediate urgency to the matter, and of course I should arrange my life so I could take the recuperation time. I left that meeting feeling particularly overwhelmed, more so, actually, than I did when I first learned of the mass.

Abba Macarius' prayer stayed with me. I prayed it holding my belly. I sang it to the rhythms of my steps as I walked. It was with me when I woke up and when I went to bed. The relief from the biopsy report was real, but steeling myself for a major surgery kept the prayer relevant.

. . . have mercy on me. Help me.

Luckily, I have friends who share a dark enough sense of humor that we could laugh about these things. One friend and I had for some time laughed together over the idea of a "weeping flash mob," a group of people who would gather in a public place but instead of dancing or playing music, would start weeping. One day, she suggested that a hospital would be an excellent place to hold a weeping flash mob. I immediately burst into laughter and said, "That would be an awesome thing to wake up to after the surgery!" While we shared a concern that I might bust my stitches laughing, I figured I was already in the hospital and they could easily just sew me back up.

Other questionably humorous thoughts before surgery included wondering if my incision, anticipated on my left side, might be a mark of the antichrist as Christ was traditionally depicted as having his side wound on the right. I eventually woke up to find the incision down the middle. By that time, we'd just entered the Easter season and so I told my friends that we would not be playing Jesus and Thomas. They were to keep their fingers out of my wound. Things like this kept me smiling through the fretting.

. . . as you will and as you know . . .

Early on April 9, my friend, Jennifer, picked me up and took me to St Luke's Hospital. While nurses came and went, inserting I.V. ports into my hand and other such preparations, we took pictures, posing as either hyperbolically scared or with thumbs up in confidence. I don't think the staff is used to their patients being quite as silly as we were, but it's among my best memories of the day.

Perhaps that is because I don't remember much else of the day. I woke up in a room and another friend, Celina, was with me. I asked her to take a picture of me, in my oxygen mask. I fell asleep as she snapped photos. She later told me that I was in two different rooms before I settled into my final room. I don't remember all the rooms.

The rest of the immediate story is anticlimactic. My hospital stay was for a full week, but I had excellent care and my pain was beautifully managed. One nurse in particular liked to laugh with me, even as she was the one who pushed me to walk and get up to speed up my release.

Once back in my apartment, friends had set up a schedule to keep food in my refrigerator. I asked visitors to walk with me to my mail box. Someone brought me the Eucharist from church. My cat loved how much I slept and slept with me. I was very well cared for.

A monk should always act as if he was going to die tomorrow; yet he should treat his body as if it was going to live for many years. The first cuts off the inclination to listlessness, and makes the monk more diligent; the second keeps his body sound and his self-control well balanced.

This brush with mortality still looms in my life. It is a dividing line. There was before the pancreatic cyst and after. Once I was able to be fully independent again, I felt as if I were in a luminous place, a particularly grace-filled time. For a story that began with "Mr. Orts, you have a mass on your pancreas," everything that happened afterwards seemed miraculous. In fact, the following summer, I created a short performance with a few friends, staging poems and prayers by mystics and visionaries. The poem I used to frame the performance is attributed to St Francis of Assisi: "Such love does /the sky now pour, / that whenever I stand in a field, / I have to wring out the light / when I get / home." The name of the performance was Wringing Out Light.

Of course, ecstatic gratitude is a difficult state to hold onto. Over the next winter, my mood dropped. The long dark nights of winter are often hard for me, but that winter seemed to drag me down farther than usual. The next spring, I was diagnosed with diabetes. Having only 60% of a pancreas meant I was no longer processing sugar very well. It has been an ongoing journey, with some rocky patches, getting and keeping the diabetes under control.

I also herniated the lowest portion of my scar, by my navel, and had to have a second surgery to repair that. Ironically, for a less invasive and dangerous surgery, that stay in the hospital was much less pleasant than my first. The most visible result of that second surgery is that I woke up to find my navel was gone. I now make Adam and Eve jokes about my belly.

Over the four years since that surgery, it stays with me, as do the Desert Fathers and Mothers. It resides in the back of my mind, this health scare and how the Abbas and Ammas, particularly Abba Macarius, were with me, keeping me focused on God's mercy and helping me laugh through it all. His prayer has receded somewhat from my immediate consciousness, and yet the world often enough reminds me it almost always appropriate to pray it.

Oh Lord, as you will and as you know, have mercy on me. Help me.

Resilience and Spirituality
by Victoria Molta

In 12-step groups, there is an expression that "recovery is an inside job." This applies to me. Turning inward and praying to God for strength and courage has propelled me forward despite the challenges and difficulties of living with a serious mental illness.

At twenty four years old, I had a mental breakdown and was first diagnosed with bipolar disorder. Years later, the diagnosis was changed to schizoaffective disorder. Schizoaffective disorder is defined as "a psychotic disorder that is characterized by recurring episodes of mood fluctuations and a loss of contact with reality." According to Wikipedia, common symptoms of the disorder include hallucinations, paranoid delusions and disorganized speech and thinking. It usually begins in young adulthood and according to the Diagnostic Statistical Manual, the prevalence estimates were less than one percent of the population, in the range of 0.5 to 0.8 percent. There is depressing evidence that social problems such as long-term unemployment, poverty and homelessness are common. The average life expectancy of people with the disorder is shorter than those without it, due to increased health problems from absence of health promoting behaviors including a sedentary lifestyle and a higher suicide rate.

The cause is a combination of genetic and environmental factors that are believed to play a role in the development of schizoaffective disorder.

Reading this information brought me back to the time of the change of diagnosis to schizoaffective disorder in 1988 after languishing on the psychiatric ward of a hospital for three months. During this time, I was desperately ill and depressed and was given the option of having electroconvulsive treatments. I agreed to it. Three days a week for several weeks, I was woken from my bed at 6:00 a.m., put on a gurney and wheeled to a stark, sterile room where I was put to sleep and woken up later in my hospital bed. Electroconvulsive therapy or ECT carries stigma with it. Most people think of the terrifying scene in the movie "One flew over the Cukoo's Nest" when Jack Nicholson's character undergoes

ECT and experiences violent convulsions. This was probably accurate in the middle of the twentieth century but by the 1980's, convulsions were slight and the patient was put to sleep.

At any rate, ECT didn't work for me. I knew that I wouldn't be able to stay on the ward for much longer than three months and was being considered to be transferred to the longer term state mental hospital. Desperate to find some way to pull myself together and re-enter the community, one day on the ward, I was given the name of a psychiatrist in town and contacted him before I was to be discharged from the hospital.

In late August, 1988, I was released. My mother greeted me with pink roses for my birthday and brought me back to the halfway house I had been living in for the past couple of years. I began seeing Dr. Klein and spilled out all of my jumbled up and scrambled thoughts and fears. He prescribed anti-psychotics, anti-manic, anti-depressants and anti-anxiety medications. The dosages made me feel constantly drowsy and tranquilized me into a walking stupor. He diagnosed me as having schizoaffective disorder and, slowly, I began recovering.

Being in recovery doesn't mean being cured. My illness was chronic with subsequent setbacks and breakdowns over the next thirty years to the present day. Yet despite this, I never lost faith in God. My spirit was stronger than my malady, like the bright sun breaking through storm clouds and lighting up the sky. I had hopes and dreams. I didn't want to give up or give in. I was given a difficult hand in my life but I chose to turn it around and give back to others.

Before 1988 and the official diagnosis, I believe I was afflicted with mental illness as a small child. I remember all the things that terrified me: doctors, deep water, dogs, cats. I carried within me profound fear and shame. I was sick and absent from school often, and my friends brought me stacks of homework papers and assignments to catch up.

My father was afflicted with a serious mental illness and he medicated himself with vodka martinis. He was a severe alcoholic who couldn't hold down a job, exploded in rages, was sadistic and objectified women. Though he was an intelligent, highly educated man who attended Cornell Law School, he never got along with his bosses and co-workers and subsequently was fired. His mother was an aristocratic, strong, narcissistic woman who couldn't understand why her son who seemingly had everything going for him-charm, intellect, movie star good looks-was such a failure. Before my father met my mother, he briefly underwent daily, intensive psychoanalysis. According to my father, the analyst advised him against getting married or having children. I never knew what the analyst diagnosed him with or why he thought my father should never have a family of his own.

Serious mental illness for me has resulted in a combination of a biological brain disease and trauma due to environmental factors. My father traumatized me with his stories of being on a train and witnessing a decapitated man's head perched along the railroad tracks when he was in the army in Germany during World War II. He told me stories about Hell and the devil who drove a speedboat in a lake of feces while unfortunate people in the water were overcome by the putrid waves. He wanted to know if his car could drive 100 miles an hour on the freeway. While drunk, he piled four of us children into the station wagon and sped to 100 miles an hour risking our lives. To say the least, I didn't feel safe or protected growing up, and my mother, a narcissist was either too busy or too overwhelmed to pick up the subtle and not so subtle nuances that were occurring in the household.

Yet, even at a young age, I was a survivor. I made friends easily though at times, I was plagued by self-doubt and insecurity. I had empathy for children who either didn't have the material things I was given or who were bullied by other children. Once, I invited a girl over to my house who stuttered and was an outcast. I tried to be nice to her and gave her my favorite treats; ripe, sweet peaches and ropes of red licorice.

I was independent and determined to learn new things though at the same time, I encountered unfamiliar situations that were very threatening to me. For example, at six years old, I was terrified of the deep end of the swimming pool at my grandparent's house. I couldn't even stand on the diving board because it was too close to the deep water despite the fact that I knew how to swim. A couple of years later, I was able to climb a high diving platform at swim school with a sweat shirt on over my bathing suit, jump off the board and swim to the side of the pool.

Though my family attended the Episcopal Church regularly, I had my own personal relationship with God. I participated in the Christmas plays, sang hymns, sat in the stiff, wooden pews, smelled the perfumed scent of incense and gazed at the colorful, intricate, beautiful stained glass windows. God showed himself to me, especially when I was afraid or when I was bullied. Once, my cousin was bullying me and I blurted out, "God doesn't like it when you say mean things". I don't know where that came from except somewhere deep inside me. I knew that God was good.

My great-grandmother, Mersey embodied God-like qualities of humility and inner beauty. She was an oil painter in her 70's after moving to California from Chicago, knowing no one, buying a house and taking college classes, showing her art to young people as an older woman. She walked through her house singing songs and tending to her pet canary "Freddy".

When she was young, Mersey met her husband-to-be at art school and they fell in love. He was a troubled man and an alcoholic. She bore him two daughters. Time passed and she realized that she could no long tolerate his irresponsible behaviors, but at a time when women didn't divorce their husbands, she did just that. She was extremely independent and set out to work at an exclusive children's clothing store in Chicago. This was also during a time when women of her background didn't work. When she reached retirement age, she fulfilled her dream of moving out west to the warm sun and scented flowers. Though she didn't attend church, her faith in God ran deep. She subscribed to a monthly spiritual publication called "Daily Word" and everyday read a new passage from it, drawing faith, hope, strength and courage from it. She was an inspiration to me.

When I was around eight years old, I spent the night at her house. She brought me to a bookstore and bought me a book of my choice. We went to the movies and I picked the movie, "The Yellow Submarine," with soundtrack from the Beatles. It brings a smile to my face to think that my elderly great-grandmother had a young soul and was open to watching a movie like that at her age. When she had to sell her house and eventually moved to a convalescent home in Connecticut to be closer to her daughter, where she eventually passed away, I was sad that I couldn't say goodbye. She left a message in me that told me that God is always present, women can be strong, independent and creative in spite of adversity or loneliness.

One last memory that I have of her was a vivid dream that came to me one night. She was sitting in a chair outside on our terrace surrounded by flowering bushes and our tremendous ash tree. The sun was out and she was warming herself. Our dog, "Roger," was walking around, his tail high, energetic and happy. As it happened, Mersey and Roger had both died within months of each other. I thought this was a sign that they were in Heaven together. It was a spiritual vision, so real, clear and different from any other dream I had.

My childhood could be chaotic with fights and loud arguments and tears within the family. There were many times when I felt alone and misunderstood. As a teenager, my older brother was deeply troubled. His bedroom was at the opposite end of the house. He locked his door and lay on his waterbed, smoking pot and listening to rock music blast from his stereo. He could be cruel and abusive. He skipped school and got into a lot of trouble. I remembered the early years and was sad because we had once shared happy memories of taking long walks in the neighborhood, cutting through people's backyards, climbing and crawling along brick walls that separated the properties.

My early years were privileged materially. It doesn't seem real to think of life back then. It was so long ago and is so far away from the simple life I live now. Though I am not wealthy, I carry rich memories and experiences that could never be taken away. Despite the troubles, I cherished life. I wanted to live to the fullest. The world in front of me cracked open like a watermelon revealing ripe, fresh, juicy, fruity flesh to savor. Yet, beneath the surface, cruelty, abuse and loneliness lingered.

Books, dolls, clothes and trips were abundant. I took tennis lessons and ballet. I was a girl scout. I was blessed with many friends in my neighborhood. I went to camp in the Rocky Mountains of Colorado. We hiked, backpacked, rode horses. The physical activities were challenging for me as we hiked miles past serene, crystal blue lakes and cantered on our horses across wide open fields. I enjoyed spending time in the crafts room making leather belts and stenciling designs into them. I made candles and decorated them with sand and seashells. I took riflery and shot at paper targets. I went to camp for two consecutive summers. After camp, I flew to Chicago to my grandparents' homes for visits.

My mother's father was vice-president of the First National Bank of Chicago and he and my grandmother lived in a big house in the upscale suburb of Kennilworth. My father's mother had inherited a very large sum of money, and her parents bought many acres of land in Lake Forest where homes were built in the 1920's for their three children. My grandmother's house was the most elegant. It was an English tudor house with vast flower and vegetable gardens tended to by the live-in gardener. There was a pool and cabana. Though often I felt alone amongst my family members, I cherished the magic of my paternal grandparent's house. There were always new nooks and crannies to discover. It was like opening a Christmas gift every day. I woke up sometimes late in the morning, walked down the oriental rug that covered the spiral staircase and into the plant filled sunroom for breakfast that Mary, the live-in Hungarian cook, prepared for me and the rest of the family. Summer days were spent in the cabana and by the pool eating sandwiches. We swam and played in the pool or went to the club for lunch. In the evening, Grandma wore an elaborate gown and we all ate by candlelight in the dining room. Mary served us dinner while Grandma, the matriarch of the family, presided over conversations. Sometimes, we went to Chicago to the University Club for lunch, to the opera or ballet or the Field museum.

When I was nine years old, my patriarchal grandparents took their four oldest grandchildren on a six week trip to Europe. I was one of the oldest and it was a grand, unforgettable adventure, one that would instill my love of travel and adventure the rest of my life.

What does my past have to do with my life today? It was confusing; privileged yet missing something; surrounded by people, yet feeling so alone. It contained seeds of love that were planted within my heart and grew to sustain me like the green stalk of a plant whose roots are embedded in an underwater stream and whose tip is warmed by the sun even when surrounded by arid, dry, desert sand. It taught me that life can be a contradiction. It doesn't always make sense. Love and hate can co-exist. Wealth doesn't guarantee ultimate happiness. It is ambiguous.

My parent's got divorced in 1976 when I was fourteen and my mother moved the five of us from our home in California to Connecticut. It was like leaving the vibrant colors of spring flowers opening up, to dismal black, white, and greys of a wintry, slushy road after a snowstorm. It was like going from a three or four dimensional world to someplace flat. My dad was left behind in California as was my best friend, Bonnie. With the passage of time, the family grew smaller and smaller. Mersey died. Then, the grandparents, one- by- one.

In 1986, my mental illness came to a head and my world shrunk. I began to live in my own world while family dropped off. The trauma of loss with its mix of hope after a storm ended, now felt like a complete, constant, blinding washout.

How did my faith carry me through my serious illness and how did courage and hope guide me through difficult times? My dad said I always had guts. He told me I am a doer, not a dreamer. I looked up the word "guts" and it is defined as "personal courage and determination, toughness of character." As a child, my mom cried on my shoulders after a fight with my dad while I comforted her. She called me her "little brick." I thought that was a strange word to use. I looked that word up too. It defined it as "fired bricks" being one of the longest lasting and strongest building materials. Bricks may also be classified as solid. I was my mom's foundation. I held her together. When my dad called me a "doer, not a dreamer", I needed to understand the meaning of that too. I assume a "doer" is opposite from a "dreamer", but I couldn't find the definition of "doer". A dreamer however is "a person who is unpractical or idealistic", a "fantasist", a "daydreamer". The antonym is "realist". I looked up "realist" and it said "a person who accepts a situation as it is and is prepared to deal with it accordingly." These definitions made sense yet at the same time did not make sense to me. It was ambiguous because I felt myself to be a dreamer too. I also felt very vulnerable and weak at times.

Mental illness is like all the lights having gone out. My world became smaller and smaller. My life became smaller and smaller. I believed I too became smaller and smaller, yet my faith in God grew larger and larger. At twenty five years old, I turned to God. I prayed. There is a saying:

> *"One day, a person walks down the street and falls in a hole.*
>
> *The next day, the person walks down the street and falls in a hole.*
>
> *The next day, the person walks down another street."*

I didn't want to fall in the same hole over and over. I didn't want to repeat old patterns. "Insanity is doing the same thing over and over and expecting different results." I had a hole in myself and I prayed to God to fill the hole. From that prayer a glimmer of hope appeared. It was a spark like a light at the end of a tunnel or someone lighting a match in the darkness. I could start to see myself coming out of the hole. I looked above me and I saw the sky, the clouds parting, and the sun. God was with me. God is with me. God is always with me. It involves an ongoing dialog with Him. He is always there. I am not alone. I began to climb up. It wouldn't be easy. I turned to others for help. I read books by people with mental illness in an attempt to understand myself. I talked to my therapist. I took medication that my psychiatrist prescribed for me. I knew that I couldn't allow myself to be in a bubble. I had to poke a finger in it and burst it in order to connect with others. Connecting to others, being genuine, asking for help are good things, not a sign of weakness. The Protestant ethic stresses individuality and independence and I grew up believing this was the sole truth. I slowly learned to trust others and hold the hands that reached out to help me.

In 1986, after years of feeling lost and alone, living in different states, and a different country, I had no sense of home. I had checked myself into the psychiatric ward of a mental hospital in Florida and left ten days later, sicker than I had ever been. I was like a pigeon I saw that had a broken wing and couldn't fly. It just looked at me blinking, as if to tell me it had no future left of flying in the sky and therefore, no purpose and no sense of joy and freedom.

My mom met me at the airport in Connecticut and was frightened by the sight of me. I was like a stranger to her. It would take years of hard work to get well. Throughout the ups and downs, the steps forward as well as the setbacks, I never lost my faith in God. I talked to God in my head, wrote to God in my journals, and kept my heart open for his will for me. I found God's goodness in people along the way whom I learned to trust and who had my wellbeing in their hearts. I had a therapist at the day treatment program I was attending who saw my strengths and intelligence and encouraged me to someday enroll in graduate school for writing. She took me under her wing. I had dinner with my mom once a week at a restaurant and she told me how important it is to have things to look forward to in life.

I was accepted into a halfway house called Interlude that had strict rules for the ten young psychiatric patients that lived there. We each had a turn to shop and cook for the other residents and counselors. We cleaned bathrooms and vacuumed floors. We volunteered or attended day treatment program or held jobs. We didn't always get along and hashed out our differences in heated house meetings. I was like a rebellious teenager testing the rules along the way. I began dating a patient at day treatment who I later learned dealt drugs and was in trouble with the police. One dark snowy night, driving my car on the highway, I crashed into a guard rail and almost killed myself. I was given an ultimatum to either break up with my boyfriend, and commit to Interlude or be asked to leave. It was like being given the option to be pulled out of a rushing, choppy river before going over a waterfall. I grasped their hands before going over the edge. I broke up with him and resumed my recovery.

1987 was a pivotal year. It was the year I chose to stay at Interlude until they deemed I was ready for a supervised apartment, and finally, independent living. I was reminded of what my mom told me, "have something to look forward to." It was also the year I met Bill. He moved into the house after a hospitalization. He had a shaggy beard and shoe laces he used as a belt. Bill was older than the rest of us. At 34, he had been through his share of traumatic events and was in recovery after many years of abusing drugs. He managed to work at restaurants as a cook over the years when he wasn't selling pot. With another chance, he was here with us at Interlude, a man, not a boy like the others. Several months later, he graduated to a supervised apartment. After several stops and starts, it was my turn to move out of Interlude and into the same apartment building as Bill. He was on the first floor while I was on the second floor.

I began visiting him at his apartment, bringing my newly adopted kitten with me. We drank coffee, smoked cigarettes and listened to Fleetwood Mac CDs. He was a hippy and had grown up at the height of that era in the 1960's and early 1970's. He played the guitar, was a vegetarian, practiced yoga and meditation and was a follower of Paramahansa Yogananda, an Indian guru who founded Self-Realization Fellowshoip. Though Bill grew up in a middle class suburb of New Haven, he was a free spirit who felt restricted within a family that didn't understand him. As a young man, he hitchhiked across the country and settled in southern California. He meditated on the beach at sunrise, cooked for his roommates and was drug-free for the two years that he lived there. It was a happy time for him until he felt the pull to go back home to Connecticut and return to drugs. Several dark years followed including failed attempts to get clean even after several drug rehabs and psychiatric hospitals. Finally, in 1987, he moved to Interlude.

At the time I was getting to know Bill better, I was dating someone else, so Bill was just a very good friend that I connected with on a soul level, though deep down, I was also physically attracted to him. I chose to push the feelings away and went on motorcycle excursions with my boyfriend Greg. Greg didn't understand me and though I liked him, I just didn't feel that he really knew me.

Stress from my job as a proofreader for a real estate magazine took its toll and my mind began to unravel once more. I broke down and ended up on the psychiatric ward of the hospital in Danbury. I suffered on the ward for three months during the summer of 1988. I was given electroconvulsive therapy (ECT) which didn't work and was a very traumatic experience for me. Psychiatric medication wasn't working and I was deeply depressed and lost.

Bill took care of my kitten and visited me in the hospital every Monday night before going to an Alcoholics Anonymous meeting. He told me that AA was the right fit that finally kept him clean and sober. When I was finally released, I told myself I would never go back to a psychiatric hospital no matter how ill I was. Checking in and out was like a revolving door of setbacks, never moving forward, never growing. I began life again at the halfway house with a new psychiatrist and a volunteer job stamping due dates into library books at the local college library.

Bill came to Interlude that fall and we stepped out on the third floor porch and held each other close while leaves on the moving branches of the trees rustled in the breeze. We found each other as if we had once known, then lost each other somewhere else in another place, at another time. We were comfortable with each other. It was like we had been away from each other for a long time and were greeting each other once again. He made me a 27th birthday dinner of shrimp and rice at a small table next to the front window of his apartment. It was the year we fell in love with each other and became a couple. The loneliness we experienced in our separate lives disappeared as we grew together.

Almost thirty years have passed since we fell in love and almost twenty four years of a happy marriage. It sounds like a cliché to say we are soulmates but it best describes who we are to each other. Our mutual faith in God and foundation of deep spirituality has carried us through serious illness as courage and hope guided us through difficult times. Bill has twenty four years of sobriety with the help of Alcoholics Anonymous and turning his will over to a Higher Power. I kept my promise not to go back to a psychiatric ward, and it's been almost thirty years since that 1988 hospitalization. Though it was one of the hardest things for me to do to avoid running to the hospital when symptoms arose, especially the first year after my last discharge, I feared if I went back into the hospital, I would never get out.

Like everyone else, life has had its ups and downs, its growth and its setbacks. Bill and I moved out of the supervised apartments in 1990 and into an independent apartment of our own. In 1993, we got married and moved to New Haven, near the town of Branford where he grew up.

I began working in the Connecticut mental health movement as an advocate and counselor. Over the years, I've marched down the streets of Pittsburgh and D.C. fighting the stigma of mental illness. I've told my story of recovery to many audiences. I've spoken to and lobbied my legislators to have housing for people living with mental illness. I've worked in mental health clubhouses running support groups for members, coordinated a peer-run public speaking project for National Alliance on Mental Illness to educate people about mental illness. I've worked on a mental health grant project as a peer mentor at Yale Program for Recovery and Community Health. I'm now working as a recovery support specialist at two housing authorities in New Haven and hope to soon resume studies for my master's degree in counseling.

Bill is retired from the restaurant business. He is a street musician with a passion for classic rock and also works per diem as a companion/home-health aide for the visiting nurse association. The sweetest thing is the home we own now and we have lived in for fifteen years. It is our sanctuary that we share with our two cats and our dog. We have found our refuge of love and safety.

Without faith, hope and courage, it is hard to move ahead in life. I never gave up even in my darkest times. I didn't walk on this journey alone. God is, was and always has been with me. The beautiful thing is that He brought me someone else whom I could love and who loves me. This gives great meaning and richness to my life.

Seeing and Being
by Wendy Devitt

It is such a challenge navigating the world and finding out where you belong, what you will do and who you will become. I have come to realize that all I have been through brought me to where I am right now, and that is exactly where I am supposed to be. One of the most transformative experiences in my adult life has been learning Iyengar yoga. The highlight of my yogic journey was meeting Geeta Iyengar in Pune India the summer of 2016. That experience enabled me to understand compassion and to learn acceptance.

This was a long journey to take, not just the flght to India but inside myself as well. There were many factors that brought me to yoga and it took some time to find the right method for me. My first experience with yoga was when I was twenty five and graduated from college. I had moved back in with my parents, and was upset that I hadn't found a job.

I experienced so much anxiety that I developed a horrible rash after graduation. When I went to the doctor to receive a diagnosis, I was hoping I was allergic to something. Instead he confirmed what I already knew, that stress was the cause of my ailment, and that he could not prescribe anything to fix it. He said that it was common after a life changing event to experience stress and that it was manifested in physical ways. He suggested I do something to relax my mind, like exercise or deep breathing.

There were other stresses in my life that had been present for many years that I did not mention to him, the fact that my eyesight was deteriorating since I was a teenager and that as a result, I was afraid of driving. It had been a tumultuous time for me living in Orlando with my parents before I left home to attend Florida State University. I always had a history of eye problems and was born with congenital cataracts. When I was very young I had surgery to remove them. After the surgery I was able to see but, I had one eye that was my dominant eye, my right eye, and my left eye was much weaker. Because of this I do not have two eyes that work together, binocular vision. However, since I had nothing else to compare my sight to, I accepted my vision as normal and did not think or realize that certain activities were challenging or could have been made easier for me. For instance when I was in elementary school I had difficulty copying from the chalk board because I was seated by a window and my eyes were very sensitive to glare. I also was a very slow reader due to having limited vison, and when I read for long intervals the words would race around the paper like ants. I didn't know that wasn't normal. I kept up with my school work as best I could but my grades definitely suffered.

I did not find out I had glaucoma until I was eighteen, my senior year in high school when my mother's insurance changed and I was sent to a new eye doctor. They did several tests on my eyes, which I never had before. One was a puff of air in the eye, which felt like someone was sneezing in my eye. The other test was a circular blue light that got very close and sat on my eye. Both tests were quite scary, and I could tell that the ophthalmologist was not pleased about the results he was getting. He told me that the pressure in my eyes was very high for someone so young. The pressure was eighteen in my left eye and forty nine in my right. This did not mean anything to me, but the doctor explained that normal eye pressure ranged from eight to twelve. He was especially concerned because the pressure was so high in my right eye, the eye I was most dependent on. He said there was nothing he could do to help, and immediately walked my mother and I to another area of the eye clinic to see a glaucoma specialist.

Before I went in to see the doctor I had to take a visual field test, which consisted of staring at a yellow dot in the center of a white screen. I was given a clicker and was suppose to click it every time I saw a light flashing around the periphery, but I was not allowed to move my eye to look for the flashes of light but, to keep staring at the yellow light in the center. When the glaucoma doctor came in, he explained that the pressure in my eye had been elevated for so long that I had started to lose my peripheral vision. I did not notice anything because I felt no pain in my eyes and still was able to read my school work and to drive. This was very common he explained since it is our central vision that we use most often and the reason why vision loss is not detected right away. Someone like me does not realize there is any change in vision until a visual field test is taken. He said that that once you start to lose vision that the sight can never be regained or repaired since it is damage that happens to the optic nerve. He said that it was like after a fire when the debris cannot be salvaged. If the pressure continued to remain elevated the result would be more vision loss. This was very serious because the pressure had already caused my vision to decrease the eye that I see out of. It was too much for me to process at one time. The doctor told me there was no cure for glaucoma, but that it could be controlled with eye drops.

I was given a prescription for eye drops with instructions to take them twice a day and return to the eye doctor to get my pressure checked the following week. The eye drops worked and my pressure went down to fourteen in both eyes.

My life changed forever that day and I have been taking eye drops ever since then to help control the pressure. Over the next three years my pressure kept incrementally going up and when it did that, I was told to take more drops. When those drops didn't work, I was given pills to deal with the pressure.

By the time I was twenty one, I had built up a tolerance to all the medication I was taking and the doctor had to zap my eye with a laser to help the fluid drain out of my eye more easily. When that stopped working he had to zap it again. I was going to the eye doctor regularly while attending school full time and working part time. I was also driving myself everywhere. One of the side effects of the eye drops was that it blurred my vision.

I wanted desperately to get out of school and to be sharing my peers's activities. So, in addition to school and work, I was also hanging out with friends late at night. Sometimes my friends would would drive to the places we went, but many times I was the one driving. My father had the idea that because I was staying out late every night that I had caused my eye pressure to go up. I was taking my drops like I was supposed to, and but when I went to the ophthalmologist my pressure was still very high.

My father thought that I had caused the glaucoma. Somehow he knew that there was a scientific connection between me going out late at night and the increased pressure in the eyes. He would yell at me "You are going to blow up your eyes!" or "You are making yourself blind by staying out late."

He said these words with such conviction that I accepted them to be true. It was so bad that when my mother took me to the ophthalmologist and the pressure was high she would ask "Could it be because Wendy stays up late?"

The doctor would say no. Staying up late has nothing to do with the increased pressure in the eye. I had advanced glaucoma, a history of congenital cataracts which was the cause for my eye condition. There was no way that I could convince my father of the doctor's diagnosis. I was unable to change his mind. Around this time I started to develop an immense sense of shame about my poor eyesight and would not ask for help when I could not see. I was living in my father's house and he had the last word. I was to blame, end of discussion.

My vision at night had gotten worse and I refused to ask anyone to drive me to work. One night I could barely see, but drove myself home because I was too afraid to call my parents and ask them for help because I feared getting into trouble. I was very uncertain of my future by living in Florida and driving everywhere.

The summer I was twenty one before I had more intensive glaucoma surgery, my parents took me to Bascom Palmer Eye Institute in Miami to see the best glaucoma specialist in Florida. He was going to put something called a bleb in my eye, which would act like a drain. I was also getting an artificial lens implant in my eye to replace my missing lens since I was two years old and meant that I would not have to wear such thick glasses anymore. My parents were very good about making sure I had the best doctors, but never checked in with me to ask how my eyesight was or noticed how bad I would squint when it was very sunny out.

The surgery required a month to regain my eye sight. I was not able to drive at all during that time. Instead I sat at home by myself during the week as my parents were at work, and my brothers were at school. I listened to music because I was unable to see the television. When, I finally regained my sight, it was not like it had been before. I was even more sensitive to the harsh Florida sunlight and my vision was not as sharp or clear as it once had been. It left me feeling very depressed and isolated because I had no one to talk to who had gone through the same experience.

I finished my associates degree when I was twenty two at the local community college. I had done some research and found that there were teachers who were trained to work with visually impaired and blind students. This seemed like a perfect job for me. There were very few schools in the county that offered this degree, but one of them happened to be in Tallahassee Florida which was about five hours away from where I lived. I took a year off from school to recover from the surgery and had one more minor surgery because I had developed a cataract on the artificial lens.

I was twenty three when I started Florida State University. While I was there, I learned so much about my own eyesight and how to better accommodate myself while I was in school. It was a fulfilling experience to learn that all of the things I had struggled with in school had not been in my mind, but just what I had imagined. I knew that I would not be able to be an independent person in Florida because eventually I was going to need to have access to public transportation.

Then I found myself back where I started after graduation, living at home. I found a job as a teacher's assistant at a nearby school. I was working during the day and like my doctor had suggested found a yoga class at the community college I had once attended. Yoga was becoming popular at this time, and I found a type called Kundalini that focused on the breath. Unfortunately, the class was held only on Monday nights. I drove myself to class and would sit with my legs crossed on the floor as the teacher explained how to breathe. There were different variations of breathing that I had no idea existed. Meanwhile, he would play Indian music in the background. The teacher was from India and always wore the same outfit, white shorts, white shirt, and sandals. His hair was short and he had a long grey beard. After the first class I left with my back feeling uncomfortable and did not feel relaxed, plus I was anxious about my drive back home in the dark. I went back the following week and the teacher had brought extra pillows for us, which made the hour long session of sitting much more comfortable. I listened to the words he was saying about connecting with our breath and I found myself relaxing to his calm voice along with the music. I noticed that I did not feel so anxious on my drive home. I had made it through five classes when the teacher came in one evening to tell us that he was going to have to end the semester early because he had to travel back to India to be with his family. I practiced sitting on a pillow in my room at home with the lights off in silence trying to recreate the atmosphere of the class. It was very difficult to do this by myself, my mind would wander and I was not able to sit still for an entire hour.

Summer was coming and there was a teaching position open at Perkins School for the Blind in Watertown Massachusetts. I applied on a whim and ended up getting the job. I was going to teach summer school and would be able to live on campus. The situation was ideal. I loved the cooler summer air of the north and enjoyed exploring the new city. What I found most beneficial was the access to public transportation. This was a new concept for me and it turned out to be most crucial as driving becoming more and more challenging for me.

I enjoyed my time so much in the summer that I applied for a full time teaching position in the fall. Just hours before I left to return home to Florida I found out that I got the job. I had lived away from home before but this was entirely different being in a new state so far away from home. I was not able to come home every other weekend like I used to when I was in college. I had not anticipated the move to be stressful. I was able to live on campus which saved money, but it gave me no real break from the job.

Once again I found myself seeking out a yoga class to manage my anxiety. I had befriended some of the other teachers and we all signed up for a hatha yoga class at a local high school. This class was different from the Kundalini class I had taken, as there was more emphasis on movement. The class was packed and I found it to be very challenging. The teacher called out the names of the poses and we followed along. I liked the physical aspect of the class but found it hard to concentrate because the class was so full.

The semester ended and I had a four week break. Around this time I was experiencing problems I had with my glaucoma. The pressure in my right eye had gotten out of control again. Once again I had endless appointments with the eye doctor and was given more eye drops. I was feeling very depressed as well as feeling guilty that perhaps I had done something wrong to cause the pressure in my eyes to go up. I knew that this was irrational, but blamed myself all the same.

I began taking three classes a week and bought a copy of Light on Yoga by BKS Iyengar. During class I was much tighter on my left side and realized how much I ignored the left side of my body due not being able to see out of my left eye. It was much more challenging for me to stretch that side of my body due to my lack of awareness.

I had become friendly with a woman at Perkins who was into holistic health and had studied yoga for several years. I had told her about my past yoga experiences and she described to me the type of yoga she had practiced, which was called Iyengar yoga. She said that I had not been introduced to yoga the right way and that this was a very systematic method that focused on alignment and holding the poses for longer amounts of time.

There was an Iyengar studio in Cambridge that she was planning to go that weekend and invited me to join her. The first thing I noticed when I got to the studio was that there were blankets for the students to sit on. This made the sitting postures so much more comfortable and I found that I was able to relax and stretch more. The next thing I noticed was that the teacher pronounced the names of the postures in Sanskrit first, and then gave the translation as well as explaining in detail how to perform the postures. There was a clear beginning, middle, and end to the pose. I do not like to wear my glasses when I practice yoga because they slide down my nose and are bothersome to me, so the verbal description of the actions made it easier for me to access them as I did not have to rely on seeing what the teacher was doing. At the end of class we ended with Savasana or corpse pose.

I was instructed to lay completely still, let go of all muscular action and pay close attention to where I was gripping. I found I had been holding tension in areas of my body that I had not even been aware of. We were instructed to not think of anything. I laid still and without even realizing it with my eyes closed I felt tears running down my cheeks. Something was happening. When it was time to sit up I felt so calm and relaxed something I had never experienced before.

Before we left I picked up a schedule of classes and knew that I would return again. I felt very sore the next day and couldn't believe that I started crying at the end of the session. I decided I would commit to a weekly class. My friend said she could not attend on a weekly class so off I was on this adventure by myself. I took a bus and two trains to get to the studio. I always got there early so I could get a spot up front near the teacher. As, I sat on my blankets waiting for class to start there were teacher assistants walking around to help. I had folded my blankets incorrectly and they showed me the proper way so that my posture would be more even. I sat slumped over and the teacher's assistant came over again and asked if she could show me how to sit so that my chest would be lifted. I did not know what she was talking about but I agreed to this. She stood behind me and placed her knee between my shoulder blades and with her hands helped to draw my shoulders back.

This adjustment was an illuminating experience as to how poor my posture was due to my visual impairment. For years I had walked with my head down and shoulders rolled forward because I was so ashamed of my eyes. When I was younger I had worn thick cataracts glasses because they did not have artificial lens implants in the seventies. This had turned into a very bad habit over the years. It felt so difficult to sit up the correct way, but I realized that my mood changed when I did it. I endured through the difficult class and looked forward to the corpse pose at the end. To my surprise I started crying again while I was lying still trying not to think of anything. On the train ride home from class I relished the way I felt. I had never experienced this before. I was calm and I could feel where I was in space. My mind also settled and I did not feel so fearful of what I was going through with my eyes and tried not to get attached to the thought of losing my eyesight but to remain in the present. I began taking three classes a week and bought a copy of Light on Yoga by BKS Iyengar. During class I was much tighter on my left side and realized how much I ignored the left side of my body due not being able to see out of my left eye. It was much more challenging for me to stretch that side of my body due to my lack of awareness.

I returned home for summer vacation to Florida and my mom noticed how my posture had improved. My parents were not happy at first that I was taking yoga because I believed that they were misinformed about that practice. My mother told me not to stand on my head, because my eye doctor had told me during a consultation that there was a vein that connected from the heart to the eyes so that I should be careful about putting my head below my heart. I assured my mother that I was taking the proper precautions. I had not realized how stressful my move to Boston had been and experienced elevated pressure in my eyes while I was there. I did not mention this to my parents when I returned home because I still thought I was to blame for my deteriorating eyesight. I was twenty six now and an adult, and figured I could handle this on my own. My visit home also proved to be very stressful because I felt some resentment towards my father for blaming me for my problems with vision, and did not feel that I could tell him what I was going through.

I had to be careful in yoga class about not doing inversions as it was counter productive in trying to keep my eye pressure down. This was another benefit to learning the Iyengar method because it is made accessible to all. My teachers would find alternative poses for me to do during shoulder stand, head stand, and full arm balance. I also noticed that my vision would be much clearer and sharper when I finished the yoga class.

On my train ride home I would relish the calmness I felt. I had also, begun writing in a journal and in my writing found myself yearning for a change. I had always wanted to move to New York City, would frequently visit Manhattan on the weekends, and I felt a need to move there. The public transportation was accessible and I had always wanted to attend Columbia University. Within the next year I moved to New York City and gotten a full scholarship to Teachers College at Columbia University to receive a Masters of Arts to further my learning of how to teach students with visual impairments. My thinking became more focused and I was able to accomplish goals that I had set for myself.

During my second year of school for my master's degree I had to have major surgery on my right eye to control the pressure. My yogic breathing helped me during the surgery which required that I remain awake. It was very scary having my arms and legs strapped down to the bed. I could see the doctors removing the old filter from my eye and watch a tube being inserted into my eye. I focused on my in and out breath and that eased my fear and allowed me to stay present. When the surgery was over my vision was compromised, and I was not able to perform the simplest of tasks like finding something in the refrigerator or dialing a phone. Before the surgery I was able to see clearly and had very good central vision, after it was like looking through a rainy windshield with the wipers broken. It was devastating for me to go from one extreme to the other in a matter of hours.

I noticed how my posture changed again, I was back to the slumped over shoulders and keeping my head down because I could not see. I was not allowed to do any physical activity for a month. I realized how yoga was now a part of my life. I didn't just want to do it, I needed to do it. It not only made my body feel good, it also controlled my mood and gave me a more positive outlook. Although I was not able to practice the postures I took my yoga mat out and practiced sitting. I sat near the wall so it was better to judge if I was keeping my shoulders back and my chest lifted.

I was able to take several elective courses at Teachers College. I took a physical education class with the idea of setting up a yoga program for visually impaired children and teens in the public school. I realized how much it had helped me to deal with my visual impairment and wanted to pass this knowledge along to others. My professor at Columbia loved the idea and so did one of my yoga teachers.

My yoga teacher encouraged me to enroll into the teacher training program at the Iyengar Institute in Manhattan. I completed a two year teacher training program and found it very challenging to keep up with the level of practice because I was teaching full time. Being in the city I found that the yoga business was very competitive and the poses I was responsible to learn did not fit into my practice. In order to be certified in the Iyengar method one has to be able to teach inversions. I worked very hard at doing this and found myself practicing postures that I should not have been doing. I made it through the first round of assessment, but when it came to the second level I did not pass. This was devastating for me and I thought about giving up on the method entirely.

However, yoga is not about reaching a certain goal it is more about the journey. After practicing for the assessment I started to experience problems with my eyes again. I had applied to study in India with the Iyengar family the summer of 2016. When I did not pass the test I contemplated not taking the trip to India. I wrote a letter to Geeta Iyengar because I wanted to learn how to safely practice poses for my eye condition. I was able to meet with her. She was very interested in hearing about my work with children with visual impairments. She also gave me modifications for the poses that I was doing. I was given the instruction to gaze downward and keep my eyes calm in the poses. This helped my poses and I did not feel the strain on my eyes like I once had. It was such an honor to meet Geeta Iyengar and have her help me with my poses. It was an amazing experience to study yoga five days a week. I had nothing to focus on but learning yoga and practicing. It is so interesting how the mind body connection works.

I found that after practice everyday my vision was much clearer and brighter much like it had been when I was younger. I even noticed that after a twisting class that Geeta taught I had a much wider field of vision and could see more out of my left eye. That lasted for about twenty minutes after class. This was my true assessment and I felt satisfied with the results.

The trip to India renewed my joy and pleasure that I had once found in yoga. The more I have learned about the yoga philosophy, it helped me discover other areas in my life that are like teaching yoga. I currently work in the New York City public schools as a teacher of the visually impaired. With my degree I am also qualified to work with families that have infants and toddlers with vision problems. It has been very therapeutic for me to help parents work with their children.

It took me many years of struggling with my visual impairment and I have found that this is exactly where I am supposed to be. My vision problems have kept me moving forward and to continue learning and just like yoga, there is not a start and finish to the path but a constant evaluation of learning what works and how to use this in order to help others.

I continue to go to the eye doctor regularly and had several eye surgeries last year on my left eye. I started to experience flashes of light and then suddenly the light that I once saw out of that eye went black. The back of my eye was bleeding. There was no medical explanation for what happened to my eye. I had to sit still for a week to see if the blood would eventually drain out by itself. After a week it was still filled with an excessive amount of blood, and the limited amount of vision I once had was still obstructed. I had to undergo surgery to remove the excess blood from the back of my eye. I had to be awake for the surgery and I relied upon my yoga breathing. I focused on my breath, remaining present in the situation and knowing that it would pass soon. A month after this happened my retina in my left eye completely detached. Over the years it had been my right eye that I had always had trouble with, and now it was my left. I was able to function fairly quickly after the surgery as it is not the eye that I depend on. However, it was a shock to go from being able to see some light and motion out of my left eye to pitch black. The doctor did not know if he would be able to restore the little bit of vision that I had. I remained calm and kept positive thoughts. The surgery was very painful and my eye was swollen shut for nine days. Miraculously the sight was restored to what it was before. I know not to take anything for granted and am thankful everyday for the vision that I have.

What It's Like To Pass Through Time After Vietnam
by Preston H. Hood III

1.

December 2011, if memory serves me right. Rock hard my heart died. My liver zeroed out, leather-fisted. Some days you don't always see the heart bleeding to marrow, hanging in the air this ache of loss above the square. Death is a channel where you tunnel through rubble.

Other times the adrenaline killing hunger that feeds me begins with Ouzo in the belly of the beast, leaning on memories like rifles. Sometimes I don't always see this dying, this twitching, manacle around my neck— the flash, Kilgore, like Arrick's suicide, or Quibbler's jump. Death's tunnel through the rubble usually strikes at dark because thought is only the electrical impulse of blood squirting; it ambushes me when I least expect it like the flash did: one instant in Na Be Vietnam, I'm jumping off a liftship in rotor whirling dust *Motha Fucka!* I-fast-run-toward curdling scream brains, bone, hair against barracks-white door I run up the stairs to him kneel over him, scrape brains blood back to… he shakes convulses hear voices: *Can save him, can save him.* hands tear-me-away. Now, I am in a in bar drinking, forgot what happened…

2.

I'd walk with morning's wind, hear its bellowing gale sweep from the north of Slievemore, back to the east, to the south into Dugort. All afternoon the sky is the dark eye of the moon. On these days I don't want to confront my demons or relive them, but I don't always have that choice, do I? After thirty years my hands tremble when I fly a kite!

Where are those days when all I had to know at seventeen was that the trains went slow enough on the long curve out from the yard, I would jump on the ladder and ride all the way to Northern Maine Junction? Where are the days at dusk when the whippoorwill calls, & the swift river is an arrow through our hearts; & the evenings, too, when we crouch on moss, shouldered between tall spruce, & listen to a moose's gruff breathing, waiting for the salt to rise like a tide to his throat? Where are the lost wails of bleating sheep calling to be found? Where is the sex we longed for & the light we hoped would transform us?

When I write in April, the sap rising, mountains stand clear & high.

Too often I remember how powerless we become beneath God's thumb

& forget how a lunar eclipse changed us while we watched

We remember the crucifix the crossing over the unattained love

On the edge near the abyss we walk a sword of life in a darker time,

and want our loved ones back

An American soldier dies every day and a half, on average,

in Iraq or Afghanistan. Veterans kill themselves at a rate of

one every 80 minutes. More than 6,650 veterans' suicides

are logged every year – more than the total number of soldiers

killed in Afghanistan and Iraq combined since those wars began.

Who listened to their darker sadness?

Who built a temple for their loss?

Lost

The thin covering between us & the world / the inward blue of our souls learning what to become / the peeling of the Asian pear from the stem outward: the precise downward spiral of the paring / blue & purple lupines that lean like Ashanti tribesman before the first freeze of autumn / the windless squall in which we see you laughing & breathing with us happily talking together on our long journey home.

Found

What we have not yet learned to do after war / zeroing in on the heart's rainbow / find a person that may make all the difference to me / listen without interrupting / know the darkness around us / the lover's moon a deeper look / enter the mist through the fire of thought & think of the thread of silence that leads to light / release the secrets we have not let go / go to the top of a trellis where light moves diagonally across the amaryllis & intersects the tips of the buds / help the child whose bird was hurt / stand against the moon like large a paper cut-out carrying the skyline / know what the dark does / listen to the white throated sparrow: *o sam peabody peabody peabody* / do the perfect dance on tree tops between light & dark / see the flicker that keeps the night awake / move into the landscape like deer or a cloud or the rain / wait for the white halos of deer heads to become spools of language disembarking souls carried away by the stars / see how the night through the measureless days furrows dreamlike before it darkens / get undressed across a room & have someone watch / let silence settle on me like snow / don't let my feelings be a barned-up bird I cannot reach / dart into the thicket like first-light finches / climb with pilgrims under a salmon-coral sky / hear voices chant invocations / rapt in a chorus of hallelujahs / whisper to the surf.

> *Fragrance of the wind:*
>
> *Sundown passing in deep woods*
>
> *Low among the stars*
>
> *Yesterday I walked about the sky*
>
> *Snow falling on blue ice*
>
> *Tomorrow I climb Katahdin!*
>
> *There many snakes in my poems but only one rabbit.*
>
> *In the attack a bullet ricochets & misses me, again.*

3.

July 17, 2017, I drove to Maine for my last cardiologist appointment. When I arrived at the Doctor's office, the nurse could not get my blood pressure after six attempts. The nurse wired me to an EKG after which the Dr. told me my heart was in atrial flutter. This after the week before when I was admitted to The Miriam Hospital Providence, Rhode Island on July 10, 2017, for congestive heart failure was a bit much to take. *Relax, take a deep breath Preston—Chill— the less stress the better for my heart.*

After seeing two cardiologists over the past five years, my new one was not only kind, but knowledgeable, so knowledgeable in fact she asked me to breathe in an out a few times holding my breath at different intervals. Then she said, "You have scarred lungs. Have you been around any chemicals?" The only chemical I have been around in my life was Agent Orange in Vietnam," I rattled off. "There could be a possible blockage in the lower blood vessels of your heart," she continued. She thought that a cardiac catheterization would make sense for me to have. Now my anxiety does flip-flops. Not to mention that my heart beats faster. Calmly, my doctor said she would schedule an appointment right away. It has been two weeks but I am sure it will happen soon.

Another bullet grazes my heart; *you lucky bastard.*

Still there are nights the moon tells me how the heart's dark repairs itself; start with a low dose of beta blocker, & over time, slowly increase the dose. I am good with that. I trust this doctor so I am learning to breathe more deeply to reduce my anxiety. Those moments: failure of the heart, atrial flutter, my anxiety heightens, entering the river of vertigo. Through my slits, through thunder heads & closed sky, crows scatter, I fall through myself like a stone, hear the rattle of the snake. Love write & save your soul I tell myself. Protect it by catching clouds in a net. Convince me in words of birds, tunes of songs; the chats of nates, the hearsays, let them go first, follow with laughter, tears. Catch them like stars eating darkness or fireflies blinking light. This is how we catch time in our hands & I have my way with it. I try to see time hold still beside me as I cup fireflies and stars in my hand. I bow with them in acknowledgment to the earth. I'm glad writing will let me live life cup after full cup. Now stir in love & kindness, tune into laughter. It's all better.

The Vietnam War by Ken Burns on PBS reveals the secrets, the lies, outrage, since the American war in Vietnam. It's a wonder that anyone still trusts this government at all. As an alumni of the outstanding "Ward 8" at Veteran Affairs Medical Center in Leeds, Mass for veterans with post-traumatic stress I hoped the PBS series would present an honest and accurate assessment of war and its aftermath. How else do we examine the somber reminder of so much loss on both sides, especially at a time when our country is more angrily divided today?"

Protest against Trump's 'fake news.' Never kill any one, anything. When monkeys speak truth, they know the cosmos. Think about it. If you see apparitions, spend a week at a Buddhist retreat. Let your heart beat in unison with another one. What more could you ask for than love & laughter swimming in a sea of fish & mystery?

To live with war is to have a word with her, when the window to the soul is open. Still there are nights I reach into the years of blackness to find dead brothers who never returned.

Today I climbed a fire ladder to the blue fruits of my passion. The moon is white like this paper. While her ribbon paths around you, the air is getting thin. My eyes probe between the darkness of thought & the grenade. I will remember your eyes forever. Tears of my sadness may never reach home.

4.

I spent seven months in Vietnam. Little did I know then that these seven months would irrevocably shape the years that followed. Whatever I saw and endured went underground. For the first ten years back from Vietnam, I thought I was fine. I had an exaggerated startle response to any noise, and I did not sleep well. When I did sleep, I would often awake in a cold sweat. I was also much quicker to anger than I had been before. Nevertheless, I led a normal life with the woman I married and was living off the land in the woods of Maine in a home I had built myself. We had a biological child, named Tanek, and two adopted children, Tamara & Arrick.

We raised them in a home without plumbing or electricity. It was a simple life but it was a good one. Off the land, off the grid was healing for me.

Curiously, more than a decade passed before memories started to surface. I'd have flashbacks; lose track of time. I would awake driving, shaking or screaming. At home my anger unleashed itself as I yelled at my wife and children. As the years went on, more memories came back and I anchored them to the page by writing them out. It was my way of trying to understand what had happened. The war had become a blur. I had very little recall of actual events. Memories came back to me, piece by piece, like a jigsaw puzzle.

I wrote part of one poem in Vietnam. With "Rung Sat" I tried to grasp the reality of this war. It was a collage of some of the search capture, search & destroy missions we had in Vietnam, and it helped me to put things in some perspective. It took twenty-five years for me to write this poem until I was finally satisfied. The poem was significant because it was the first time I was honest with myself about what I had done. That poem served as witness in my chapter: The Poem That Was Snake Medicine. Sherry Reiter, editor and author of Writing Away the Demons, Stories of Creative Coping Through Transformative Writing, with contributors, put it this way: *It is said that poison can be ingested, and if one survives, it is possible to transmute the toxins. Preston is absorbing and integrating the poison, rendering it less toxic with each poem he writes. He is performing one of the most difficult of all transformations; the conversion of blood to ink.*[1]

I watch someone carry packages to a friend. I shout & jump straight up into intervals of time until we can meet again. Every direction a flake of stone, a bit of luck.

You're nude, I'm hard. Pinch my nipples with your fingers. The echo of romance leaves its shadow as a cocoon. I learn to hold my fist as my heart. With unfulfilled love I have found another. So many things press into the heart, the interactions of this world, the earth turning against the cobalt-etched light. Eyes probe: Questions remain. Are all men brothers? What went wrong? And my marriages, too? The undertow will carry me to the fathoms. Living alone on North river I will figure it out.

An opening in the sky: before the dead crawl out I stitch it up with the white line of my thinking & watch the sunrise.

The uncoupling of my first marriage happened while we stacked the wood & planted the green beans; it happened over the White Christmas with name embroidered stockings & wooden toys we made for the kids. It happened in the silence of our bed without sex. Thirty lifetimes ago we burned candles in our house of love.

And in my second, what happened with the vocabulary between us, this thin covering between us & the world? Sometimes it was the inward blue of our souls learning what to become. Other times I held her before me able to love all of what I had then. In all honesty, I believe we still love each other, but we could not make it work.

Somehow, I will emerge having felt & learned & thought deeply; I will follow the path of my own heart On this path I will walk for miles.

5.

After all these years killing still peels back memory like flesh. I watch the dead rising. The planet I live on drops a grenade at our feet. I will rebuild the architecture of my losses. At dusk I will hear the chirping of birds with the water falls in the stones & ravines & distant streams. This evening the red moon may eddy on the pond.

Hell week, & it's not over yet…

Sunday night we know the bull horn bastards are coming, but we don't know exactly when until we hear the barracks door slam against the metal locker, and startle us awake. Like obscene beasts from your childhood, three men assault us, smashing bats against a metal trash can, shouting, "Wakee, wakee, rise and shine, the Chief's in the alley, your ass is on the line. All slipknots hit the deck and get your asses outa the bunk. You'll think quick, when we get through with you. Nuts to butts to the grinder." So begins the training that molds the rest of my life.

How Pavlov's dog relates to our harassment is this: From the moment we begin we're conditioned by the whistle. "So maggots, listen quick," scream the instructors from megaphones three inches from our ears, " One whistle means hit the deck, two whistles, attention, three whistles, crawl." The guy next to me mumbled something under his breath. Instantly, an instructor was screaming three inches from his face. "When we say jump, maggot you say how high? Hear me?" "Yes instructor," he shouted back.

We're all assholes and elbows, either hitting the deck, or at attention, or crawling around. What a circus of numb sculls we are. Whistles at the left of us, whistles to the right, always whistles in our face. At times we barely knew our ass from a hole in the ground.

Of course, hell had its way with us, the whistles were high pitched squeals blasting faster than we could react. We were all howling dogs, fucked up as Hogan's goat lost in a maze. I looked like three people in one frame going in different directions at the same time. An instant seemed to last forever, evolutions of running, swimming never seemed to end. The blur of time: the cold shivering of your teeth rattling in your brain. The fire hose water gushes against me & flattens me to the road. My face frozen face, raw-red; tears freezing in five degrees. I thought, most of us barely knew the score. They called this appreciation wet suit swims. "Yea, better get used to it.."

Of course, we always swam them in fatigue greens. We knew by now not to whine.

I remember I'm running, falling & pushed along, wads of spit frozen on my lips as I hit the pavement. Here I am, headlong and half-awake, in a frozen stare of stumbling ahead on a perimeter road somewhere, barely keeping up to the pack, soaked, frozen like a blow-up doll. Sometime before, we were hosed down & drenched with water, flopping around like otters on an ice slab. Our bulging K-Pok-life jackets over green fatigues, were crucibles sinking us down. It was bad enough trying to figure out how to put on the crap, let alone run with the sodden weight. Everything is against us, the bull horns blaring: "Maggot, asshole, scumbag, you'll learn to like cold, or if you want, take a warm shower, have a steak dinner then it's back to the fleet." We've been running for what seemed to me forever, one hundred & fifteen of us. Before we left the barracks, bullhorns screamed in our ears: "look left, look right where ever you look, thirty of you won't last the night." *How cheerful*, I thought. By now, I was so far at the end of the run, I could barely see the other guys ahead of me in the dark. Then a bull horn voice blared at me, "Hood, hit the deck, give me twenty push-ups. Your so fuckin' slow you could make a freight train take a dirt road." I was slow doing the pushups. Suddenly, I was lifted by a boot so far up my ass that my balls ached when my face hit ground, my red helmet driven into my forehead, when the strap broke "What the hell," I said. But it was too late. The instructor jumps on me, like stink on shit. "Hood, keep your filthy trap shut, hit the deck & give me twenty more. You can pretend it is your mother below you or your girlfriend or whoever it is that you want to fuck, just don't whine again if ya know what's good for ya."

How far we have run or how long seems irrelevant. I think I hear splashing ahead, and some guy saying, "What the fuck? Are you shitting me, you want me to go in there?" All I can see was a kick and a splash then another kick and a splash, one body after another wallow in. I heard another guy yell out, "I'll quit before I swim in a cesspool of shit," then he throws his red helmet down so hard it cracks against the cement pump cover and walks away. By the time I reach the pool of floating turds & piss, the smell is so over whelming, I gag & puke. I didn't even think about it; my mind in neutral, my ass in gear, I dive in head first, swim as fast as I can to the other side, but there are too many of us in the cesspool, we slow each other down. Finally, one by one after one by one, we crawl out on the icy edge. Like penguins in an oil slick, we slip, & slid, shit-smelling wet, shivering to the ground, we are on our feet again stumbling, running the best, we can trying the hell not to fall.

On the night road back were guys walking without helmets and shivering, all of us colder than we ever felt. Then those prick bastard instructors only give us a two- minute cloths drop shower, a one minute clean up, dry clothes, a warm coat & zero minutes to rest. The instructors are back batting the galvanized trash cans, screaming at us to crawl out to the grinder get hosed down, divided into 6 men & an officer per boat. We are back in the saddle again, carrying our loaded duffle bags heading to the beach with our inflatable boat smalls (IBS's) driving our helmets through out heads

6.

Especially in the night raid on June 1970 at Ham Long District area (Kien Hoa), when he discovers one VC team, he waits calmly for the enemy moving in the ambush position – kills 3 VC and captures important documents.

In minute variations of thought my nightmare see-saws on an iron pipe fulcrum, I fall, fall. I fall into sleeplessness, tension, anxiety where my words torque in thought & the ghosts of war flash back: *Bullet thru her head, a knife slits his throat, blood gushing out. A drowning. Memories like fallen rock plummet thru my head. A hyena's cry heard thru a scream.*

In Nam I blast a bullet through her skull. I slit his throat. Agony's halted scream. So deep inside me, arrows strike my heart. Blood clogs the brain.

The Viet Cong girl approached with grenade raised in her hand ready to throw. Deaths rattle in my ears— my M-16 blew out her face… Rain across Buddha's folded arms… The war continues to flank me… Her ghost winters in the chunk of my unkempt head where I can't suture the distance between sadness & death… Why didn't we care beyond the river of blood if we leveled the place. We unleashed ourselves like venomous snakes.

Does the spirit ever rise from war's raw shout of brains blown out? I leave one place for another & never arrive.

In morning the sky swirls crimson, tries to seek its shape. The moon clouds. I live with someone's pounding fist.

In time, maybe, I'll see a glorious shaft of light! Become a tree toad!

7.

Look! I see Arrick's smile in Sundog's reflective ice.

I think the moon silver. The sky clears. My heart pumps its blood.

I toast to life I toast to life

Recline. Observe. Appreciate.

Herring-bone clouds disperse

In sky.

What shall I share between us today?   A journal entry? Haiku?

At White River Junction VA the PTSD (Post Traumatic Stress Disorder) Veterans on the way to Ground East are like aching teeth in the VA's jaw. Flash backs reoccur, no intimacy— the bones of their shadows not yet wormed. For us the war wages on, a blood mark years-long. Human beings who once lived among us not yet reborn.

8.

Yes, I am happier living with humans & goats, not celestial bodies. I still want the touch of love: my time will arrive when the amaryllis intersects the tips of the buds then & only then you can give me an updated analysis of finally coming home.

What comes next after the rainbow, the luminous slant of light is the flat calm of pond stillness where a frog trills a single note & the sound of the oriole older than anyone. We assume the spirit lives to a renewal, yet we enter the abyss and find no answers. The most damaged of us struggle with belief. We want our loved ones back & learn the best part of our singing are the shadows we leave as we travel this earth, climb from our struggle into the marvelous. Meteor across October's turning colors. A good omen.

Writing through blood-pigment-loss, the granite wall of grief, this weight of years measured by suicides, of snows clinging to the soul, & the shooting-car-crash of my son by his own hands was as if he helped death scrawl her own name with lipstick beside his across the bathroom mirror. Here the landscape darkens knows more than I know. Really?

I don't know about you, but as winter's tubers shoot-up like red-asparagus, the peonies in the south garden push the need-to-be-raked leaves aside, & my juices begin to flow. I'm fed-up with the Four Horsemen of Apocalypse riding headless through darkness, luring me into their stalls.

Between silence & shouts, the promise of twilight before first light, against the orange sun, I see green show up again, & the garland bough opens my heart to singing: from dark to brown, from shady green to deeper jade, my vein-like leaves are hues, while the chlorophyll tone of lightness raves from that open branch of sky. Beyond these words, this random timbre of light, quiets me. Such an up-lift of memory. This piano of cloud where dreams are born—luminous tinge!

Look with me now: the stars that pulse like beacons. It's raining snow, & the evening is a wildness of love. The roof does not leak, & the wash of moonlight through the skylight is a moment of passion that wants you. Sit with me until dawn. Open our wounds to rain's forgiving shades, let the sea wash our hair & after, listen to the minnows breathe in shoals. Minnows breathe in shoals.

At sixteen I wrote: *hell is in shell as he is in she.* Hormones raging. At seventy-four I wrote: a poem, "beauty is a cardinal." At sixteen I cried, I was sad, I was a winter full of icicles. Now I think back to when I was nine almost ten, I'd I lay awake listening to my parents argue. I was dragged down stairs by my shrieking-drunk mother, "You're no damn good, like your father who just bolted out the door, screaming "fuck you" at my mother. This happened for years over and over and over. Then she would pass out and I would cover her, go up stairs, get a few hours sleep then wake and make breakfast for my sisters and me, and get them ready for school. Needless to say that by the time I arrived at school, I was a basket case and a screw-up. No wonder I was depressed. How I manage to do this all those years until I was seventeen, I don't know, but I did.

What is important here is that I remember asking myself, who I was and where I was going in my life? More recently, taking part in a documentary film: Hunter in the Blackness, Veteran's Hope and Recovery, I said even with all the childhood abuse, I found that walking in nature is good for the soul. And when my parents would ship me off to my grandfather, I had glimpses of calmness when my grandfather would walk me in his back woods through the log cutters camp then to his open hay fields where he would sit with me on a stone wall and I would listen to his stories when I was five. Thinking about this almost three quarters of a century later, I thank my lucky stars for my grandfather, who was more like a father to me than his son was a father to me.

I remember this particular day more clearly because this day, Gramp, taught me how to whittle a piece of wood. He showed my how to open a knife and push the blade along the wood away from me. I was in my glory. I noticed he had turned the other way and I just kept whittling for awhile then I stopped and tried to close the knife, but that did not work out so well because I closed his knife across my finger. And it was bleeding, and I was scared because I thought he would yell at me like my parents would when I did something wrong. Just as Gramp turned back from looking across the field I quickly put my bleeding hand behind my back, he spotted the blood drops across the rocks, his hand hopped along in the air, his forefinger plunging at each bloodspot drop. What I did not realize then was that he was making a game out of it for me. His finger finally stopped behind my back when it found mine bleeding, and he asked, addressing me as "Old Timer" which made me feel like I was an adult too, "How did you cut your finger?" as he immediately wrapped my finger with his handkerchief to stop the bleeding. Hesitating, "I closed the blade on my finger," I sheepishly answered. Not even yelling, Gramp responded, "That was not your fault Pret, it was mine. I did not show you how to close the knife correctly."

I always remember this story because it was the first time I was not yelled at by an adult. As I grew up in life I always remember this story; it gave me some perspective that there was more to life than yelling. For the first time I was not afraid. Love from my grandfather was unconditional. This single experience always stood high above my youthful wrong doings with which my parents always put me down. No wonder, Seal Team training and "hell week" raised my self-esteem.

Now, seventy years later, I have realized that sounds and breath in poetry and breath in my practicing of Yoga Nidra Meditation by Richard Miller, Ph.D., along with a class of Conscious Breathing are helping to heal my heart and my soul. All I have to do is be open to both and love will follow.

In the woods of Maine while living off the land and off the grid with my family, I tried running marathons to ease the tension in my mind of war and conflict. For twenty years the "runners high" seemed the answer, but eventually I realized that the more I worked (aversion) and ran, my anxiety would end. Not so, my body, my hip, and now my heart were telling me something different. Still the search for my own truth was not being answered, and my inner conflict remained unresolved. Happiness seemed to be a hidden landscape I could not find no matter how I pursued it. I could send my "healing thoughts" to others, but for myself I could not do the same.

Besides I had been at this a long time. At sixteen, after years of parental put-downs, I questioned myself even more, who am I to live in the shadow, how could I be a man with this baggage? I sought negative attention because I was getting no positive attention at home. I had nothing to lose, but I was afraid. Why should I be fearful of these thoughts, these questions? Looking back after all these years later, I lived in fear of a state of constant arguing, yelling and tension: was I going to be just like my parents in my life's journey on this walk? Thinking this led to my teenage depression.

But somehow two realizations happened to me at this time. For what ever reason, I started writing, and it made me feel darn good. Secondly, I somehow realized not only did I need intellectual stimulus, but also I needed to play a sport to ease my thoughts. Even though I figured this out on my own. I was still not totally aware of the breath & depth of emotions being expressed. I sought out sounds and sayings in my disguised vocabulary of a profane language I invented to swear at teachers. At the time I did not know as Keith Wilson the Korean War Veteran, Naval Academy man, and New Mexican poet was well aware of: "What is the relationship between my breath rhythms and my heartbeat? Am I truly conscious of my body I write out of?" Of course, I was completely unaware of my emotional vocabulary. That, as Keith says, "constitutes the language of my dreams and my most inner inexpressible thoughts?" Do I inhale the breath of a poem I should write? Am I truly aware of the world that seems to surround me? What do I really think of the world?"

A few notions seem realistic to me now, of why my emotional self waned. I was too busy raising my sisters in an inferno of enduring put downs, how could I be aware of my breath, rhythms and heartbeat. On top of this, I was too immature, and had only read two books in high school: A Weed in the Garden, and Black Beauty which doesn't get me too high on the totem pole of life.

It seems when I figured out that the older I got, the more it was people that are most important, people's feelings, and how we communicate. Take technology and throw it away, put two people by the campfire face to face, and they have to talk to each other.

Lately my river of energy is surging, and I am more at peace since discovering Integrative Restoration (iRest) Yoga Nidra Meditation, a program for healing PTSD by Richard Miller, Ph.D. Besides it is a proven effective approach to using Yoga Nidra Meditation, and deep relaxation techniques to overcoming trauma. I was introduced to iRest Yoga Nidra Meditation by Scott Cornelius, Ph.D. At Ward 8 at the Central Western VA Healthcare Facility in Leeds, MA He encouraged me to take a course to facilitate it by volunteering at Ward 8 and the YMCA. I am a Level 1 teacher of its practice.

According to Richard Miller, "Yoga Nidra allows you to be in the present moment, accepting everything as it is, no need to change anything. This patient practice brings success, and bears its rewards with love and right action. Stop judging yourself, learn to be welcoming. Know that every thing is a messenger, know you are always doing your best. Understand the law of awareness. Discover your non-separate wholeness. Practice little and often."[2]

It did take me about four months to decide to do the practice because over the past year, I have been going through some major events that have changed my life: my second divorce, moving to a new place, buying a home, the deterioration of my hearing, and my rapid-fire atrial flutter, and inactive sarcoidosis of my heart. Considering all this and the amount I had to do on the fix-up project of my house, I finally determined the time where the benefits out weigh the negatives. When I think back on my life again, it all comes down to breath (pun intended). Lately I have been thinking of my heart, my breath patterns, my dreams, my inner most self. They discovered sleep apnea when I was tested; it turned out very severe. I had thirty nine apneas per hour. Now with a C-PAC machine, I am down to two per hour with a good night's restful sleep.

Just yesterday I completed a four week course in Conscious Breathing taught by Carol Pedigree who believes our mind and body are not separate but are one in function. Just think, explains Phil Nuemberger, Ph.D. in Freedom From Stress, "We have not breathed normally or naturally since we were babies, allowing our breath to massage our organs. In moments of stress we breath through our chest not our lower diaphragm. In moments of stress we are not getting enough oxygen in to our blood stream which puts a strain on the heart."[3]

Again I claim that walking in the woods and mountains and fields massages the soul and since I have moved to the East Branch of the North River in Colrain, MA, I feed the birds their daily meals, just watching them share their seed with the squirrels is another way to massage my heart. Truly even with all my heart issues, only this past year has my heart and soul soared while living with these companions on the wooded-pine river. I have counted up to a dozen species sharing food together. On Arbor Day a white throated sparrow sang, O Sam Peabody, Peabody, Peabody, the river narrowing into a V like geese flying; it holds a nest of red-winged blackbirds finding comfort with the shadow fish when our voices rise and lower with the current. Downriver, on the southern arm of my property on the island two cranes reach out and up as they lift their winged shadows, like flying stilts, into the bleached clouds, black skies forming a darkness above us. And a week ago Ground Hog day of course he sees his shadow again this year. It is no surprise nearing zero, a tribe of morning doves flood the feeders, and a pair of male female cardinals share their corn and sunflower seed with a flurry of black-capped Chickadees that just flocked in from the sumac tree. Here five Blue Jays swoop down in argument of protest to attack the feeders. Yes, this is truly winter, but not as lonely as it could be without their company. And this too shall pass into spring nestled with the peepers; a frog trills human history in a single note, a high lyric meditation. It is this that allows the soul to migrate from its struggle into the marvelous. With the influx of light summer will arrive in due time with this uplift of memory. How can we not know the best part of birds singing?

Today is the best part of the winter season when I read surprisingly great news that I receive about my hearing dog, Gilmore, a black lab will I come to training to meet her at the end of the month. This time my heart is in a good flutter of excitement and joy, while at the other end of the phone I hear her bark in the wind of my knowing we will soon be companions for life. I quiver like a voice giving way to ecstasy, a sound disguised as a flute, a distant moan streams in, but only for a nanosecond my world appears beautiful, as luminous streams fjord in from the sky. Today, my heart is an orchid, tomorrow a red-tinged sunset., twilight an evening mist of stars—a dream come true. I hear luscious rain through the dark, rising up, falling… What else is there but to see the moon enter midnight's human hum through the bird feeders and the patio outside.

People say things happen in threes and for me they have: my practice of Yoga Nidra Meditation, the completion of my Conscious Breathing class, and this ultramarine gift of Gilmore are blessings. Thankfully, at the end of my life is a beginning, the river below my house is steel blue while the geese across the twilight honk. Today, I am not tied to the dark by ghosts, neither is Gilmore. Some day while we walk, our spirits will rise haze over marsh, ultramarine. It seems to be true then that my happiness will come by me accepting everything just as it is., not changing a thing. As Jean Klein states, "Make the practice your own."

NOTES

1. Reiter, Sherry. "Writing Away The Demons; Stories of Creative Coping Through Transformative Writing," *North Star Press of St. Cloud*, 2009.

2. Miller, Richard, Ph.D. "Yoga Nidra; A Meditative Practice for Deep Relaxation and Healing," *Sounds True, Inc.*, 2010.

3. Nuernberger, Phil, Ph.D. "Freedom From Stress, A Holistic Approach," *Hamalayan Institute Press*, 2007.

The Spirituality of Older Women
by Maria Bernardi

When we think of spirituality, we do not include older women because despite the great changes that paved the way for women to become leaders and participators in business and politics they continue to face inequality. We still live in a patriarchal society, and one with little respect for older people.[1]

Many years ago, when I came down with a chronic illness, yet persisted in teaching because I hadn't yet accepted the change, I received an invitation to attend a conference of the Cherokee Nation. At my college I was teaching European Governments as well as International Relations so when I arrived in Talequah, Oklahoma, I found myself learning about a new culture in compressed time. While I felt that my world was changing beyond recognition because of my extreme fatigue, another one opened up that would absorb me for the rest of my life, as well as being a special gift that would guide me through my illnesses.

The conference was a revelation to me. At the airport a friendly blond woman was waiting to drive me to the conference that identified herself as a member of the Cherokee nation. Startled, I asked her to explain. She replied that she was one sixteenth Cherokee and thus given the option to remain a member. She and her husband were eager to do so because, "We have children and I know that they would be very well cared for by the People if anything happened to us."

At an afternoon session on women and spirituality, I met the presenter, a Cherokee poet and writer, Awiakta, and, as we talked afterwards, I struck up a friendship with this imposing person with raven hair and a ready laugh. We spent the following afternoon together sharing our thoughts as if we had known each other all of our lives. We discussed our beliefs on the importance of cooperation, mutuality and caring in society. Both of us felt that a spirituality that didn't inform personal and social relations with deep respect was of little value. I was filled with admiration for the way in which Awiakta carried out her work on behalf of her people, without any self -promotion. In that short period of time she introduced me to a culture where older women have primary roles and to a way of life with differing views of time, history and spirituality.

The conference was organized by the well- known leader of the Cherokee nation, Wilma Mankiller. The presentations were given and attended only by women. Just a few Cherokee men showed up and they sat quietly in the back row.

The Cherokee people revere the Corn Mother. She has taught them about the spiritual meaning of corn, about strength, balance, adaptability, cooperation, unity in diversity, centered in the law of respect and also that everything is interconnected. They believe that every living thing is sacred and governed by the laws of relationship.[2] The Corn Mother is revered as the grandmother who teaches that harmony, not dominance, is what matters and that she is the life force, the Spirit that unites all things. Every Indian nation reveres her, whether Hopi, Ojibway, Wampanoag, Chickasaw, or the Laguna Pueblo, and each of them includes a woman also known as the Clan Mother and the Faith Keeper.

I have always felt a profound faith. But the illnesses that transformed my daily life helped me to renew and deepen that faith. That spiritual renewal was inspired by the fact that I was now experiencing a very different way of being as I could no longer pursue the busy schedule of teaching and social activism. I remember emptying my office and putting a life I loved in boxes of syllabi in the attic. It was also a time when my husband was working incredible hours with a start up company and I found myself struggling by myself. But over the years, my solitude left me room for reflection, providing an opportunity to appreciate the beauty and mystery of creation, as well as the blessings in my life, almost as if I had been granted second sight. I found myself open to experiences that in my former healthy life I would have passed by, as I rushed from one task to another. Just as cosmologists are discovering new dimensions in our universe, there are more levels of personal awareness than we are open to.

Among the issues I face from living with Interstitial Cystitis, a neurogenic illness that affects my bladder and immune system, are Chronic Fatigue and Fibromyalgia, meaning often searing attacks of pain at night and tiring very quickly during the day from what seem like ordinary chores. Fibromyalgia has made it difficult for me to walk or to stand for a period of time, and I found it humiliating to be on a wheelchair because of the long lines before security at the airport. However, since I couldn't get any medical help when I first came down with it, I found a book on my illness that was more than useful because it helped me discover that walking is actually healing. I now walk for a mile almost every day in good weather and it has made a great difference. Interstitial Cystitis means that I have to get up at night several times. But over the years, I have learned not to tense during attacks of pain, but rather to relax and engage in something that will take my mind off of them.

Although I now live without routines I can count on, needing to constantly rewrite my daily life, my passion for human rights is still an important goal for me. I even found that passion enlarged, and became concerned with the social images and the rights of the disabled as well. My first experience in becoming an advocate for the ill happened spontaneously. In the early years of my illness when I was still able to travel for my work, I gave a presentation at a national conference of hospice workers focused on grieving, based on a book I had written. While at a social gathering before the proceedings, I heard a priest referring to the "unfortunates who are ill." Although we became friends, that remark sent me back to my hotel room where I tore up my presentation and wrote a new one. The following day, I spoke not only about allowing oneself to experience the turbulence of emotions around loss, but also about my personal experience. "Perhaps one way to create a common social discourse is to think of ourselves as not only defined by our careers or social roles, however necessary these categorizations are, but also as members of a circle of being, held together by a web of common experiences and possibilities. In my struggles as a person who is ill, I discovered that the line between illness and health, good luck and bad, is a very thin one. If we recognize ourselves in those who suffer, we can heal ourselves and our society." I also talked about the importance of anger in the process of grieving, not as wrath directed against oneself or against others with the intention of causing harm, but as a healthy aggression leading to inner transformation and empowerment.

In our society, illness is commonly viewed as a physical problem, ignoring the many ramifications of physical suffering. These often include grief, emotional upheavals and the search for meaning. We are also unaware of how many people acquire the qualities of wisdom, forebearance and compassion on their difficult journey.

When we think of the word healing, we envision physical remedies. However there are many aspects to healing. Finding comfort in a metaphysical and spiritual sense in a world that seems terribly unjust is one of the most important aspects of our journey on this earth. Another way of improving our lives is by creating a social discourse that brings us out of the isolation that our physical problems impose on us. We become part of community again, rather than being marginalized. An important part of recreating our lives is finding new ways of contributing to society. Each one of us has the capacity to attend to the heart, mind and spirit. Thus we can all experience improvement in our situations whether or not we can be physically cured. Most of all a loving presence is an ongoing form of healing.

After I had been diagnosed with my chronic illnesses, I found that my circle of friends diminished. Except for a few of my former colleagues, most of my friends stopped calling and when we do meet occasionally, my condition is not part of the conversation. That experience inspired me to study how language is shaped to exclude many people from the broader society and also to realize that in a society that emphasizes health and fitness people have a great fear of vulnerability, mortality, and differences.

In the broader society, the dominant world is that of the healthy. When I pass through their corridors I am invisible. It is not surprising for both worlds have such opposite frames of reference and there is no bridge of common experience or discourse for our separate realities. It is as difficult for a healthy person to imagine the exhaustion that I live with as it is for a person who lives in a tropical climate to see him or herself shoveling snow on a January morning.

Conversations flow around and through me: friends speak of

how wonderful they feel after their daily jog around a pond or after a few hours at a gym. Sometimes they will complain about fatigue if they have been working too hard of if they have had a wakeful night as if the good health they radiated were an entitlement. When I listen to people complain of difficult nights and what seem to me as minor problems, I have to remind myself that everything is relative, that for someone who is always feeling well, a sudden discomfort is upsetting.

"You look wonderful," acquaintances assure me when I am not feeling well and thus obliterate me with that one sentence. That phrase is meant to console me as well as to create a distance from my situation. It took many years for me to understand that fear rather than indifference is the reason so many people avoid the subject of physical problems. "They just don't get it," is a phrase I repeatedly hear from friends who have disabilities. Understandably it is difficult for people to imagine the hard work of accomplishing the slightest thing. There is neither a discourse in our society for such situations, nor accepted patterns of behavior. Illness occurs out of sight in hospitals, outpatient clinics and doctors' offices, but not in society.

We fear what appears as weakness. We especially fear that illness is contagious, however unreasonable that might be or perhaps it is the vision of the human condition that we wish to blot out. Ironically those of us who are ill or grieving always feel that we should protect others from our reality or even console them. I find myself assuring people that I manage very well because I do not want pity, and because of a taboo against upsetting others.

As a result I began to pay careful attention to the way I spoke and to coach my family on ways of conversing with me. My husband has learned to say, "I am so sorry for what you are going through," when I traverse a difficult period. Such an acknowledgment is really all I need. I also found a way to reply to the social exchange of "how are you," with the expectation that I will answer, "Just fine thank you." Instead I simply answer, "I am."

I found myself with losses and gains intertwined, experiencing how what once seemed like small events touched my life. The cousin of a Mexican friend of mine came to Boston with her little daughter who needed heart surgery. I wrote to the little girl, Ybi, sending her the pop-up cards children love and telling her she had a grandmother in the United States. When Ybi recovered and the family left, her parents wrote me a long letter including a beautiful photo of five-year-old Ybi with long black hair and an enchanting mischievous smile. On the back her mother wrote, "With much affection to my grandmother, Marguerite whom I will always remember as someone special in my life." Her mother's note spoke of the loneliness of sitting on the 17ᵗʰ floor of Massachusetts General Hospital in an alien country whose daughter was in the hospital. Then there was my private exchange with my friend Humaria from Pakistan who told me that the FBI was watching them although her husband was a successful businessman, and when I told her about my insomnia she sent me a prayer with a note, "Just put it under your pillow." These moments would not take a large place in the lives of the healthy. But happening within such a short time made me reflect that there is another level of awareness we pass by in our hurried lives, a level that knows no time or geography and where we are instruments of consolation, speaking to each other in the secret recesses of our beings.

In the first few years of my illness, I was drifting, trying to reshape my life. Then, just by chance I heard about a new Women Studies Program at Brandeis that was accepting women from outside the university. When I became a Scholar at the Women's Studies Center for Research, there were only six of us, but now there are over eighty and it is housed in a special building. It is a place where being multidisciplinary is not a political issue and I could write in many areas. Fortunately, one of my passions was writing books and I no longer had to do this late at night after a day at work, and household chores. Writing and doing research became my new life and I wrote one book after another in different fields; poetry, women and human rights, and even a book to bring some understanding of how to relate to people that have health problems and reveal that they can have interesting lives. But I cannot participate fully in events at the Women's Studies Research Center; am unable to go to the artists' retreats where I traditionally worked on my poetry; can no longer go out to visit friends, or to a concert -- everything which once nourished my soul, so I have been continually creating a new life for myself in many different ways.

In 2016, a Wampanoag Tribal Councilman opened the Radcliffe Institute's Native Peoples' Conference with a blessing. His blessing was then clarified by reminding people that Harvard's nearly four-century presence on the Banks of the Charles has been a thoroughfare for his people for over 12,000 years. He spoke about the dignity of his people that needed to be defended. As someone who follows and admires their path, I did not sue the physicians responsible for the four medical errors I experienced in the past few years that made my chronic illnesses seem like mere headaches. One of them was a severe brain injury eight years ago that would have killed me if my husband had already left for Paris to be with his family because I was lying unconscious on the bathroom floor and hemorrhaging in my brain. It was caused by a medication that no one with very low blood-pressure such as mine should ever have taken. An ambulance took me to a nearby hospital that was unable to care for me so I was sent to one in Boston. I remember three physicians coming to see how I was every few hours that night. A week after I was released, I had an appointment to discuss the results and was told, "You have lost your short-term memory and your left lobe is permanently damaged." When I left, I was in tears. I am a right and left brain person, and the left brain is where the subconscious resides and kept me writing every day. I was not offered any medical help, but my daughter immediately sent me a series of visual puzzles to help me regain my concentration, and a notebook computer to help me take notes during my research. Struggling with short-term memory is a problem that few people are aware of.

Another medical error has robbed me of my sleep, and I often experience nights with no sleep at all, or with just two or three hours. Years ago, my daughter who lives in London, was going through a more than difficult period. Since I didn't have the stamina to fly over and spend time with her and was more than worried, I was unable to sleep. A social worker referred me to a psychiatrist who could give me medications to help me through the night. I knew nothing about drugs or sleep aids. I am very thin and don't weigh much, but I was told to take six Xanax a night. When

I started going down to four and then two, I started hyperventilating and having anxiety attacks. What I didn't realize was that I was experiencing the symptoms of a drug addict on withdrawal. It took me some months to find an appropriate physician to help me. He worked out a plan during our meeting that proved helpful in getting off a medication that is very addictive and a prescription to help me sleep that unfortunately had too many side affects for me. What remained was an inability to sleep. I used to sleep ten hours at night and two in the afternoon because of Chronic Fatigue. Since I love doing research and have worked in so many different fields, I read about the results of addiction and found that it changes a person's brain.

Ironically, "the opioid crises" is now a national issue, which means that I can't take what I need to help me sleep because physicians have to follow strict rules for sleep and pain medications. Also with the brain of someone who was addicted, I need to take three instead of two pills for sleep and I have only three medications that are helpful even though they only work every twenty one or twenty five days. I have tried homeopathic remedies such as valerian, but they have not proved helpful. I keep a log of each night, of hours slept and medications taken. When sleep eludes me, which happens very often, I go into another room and read a book for a few hours. The following day is like climbing a very steep mountain, but I have always loved reading my way around the world, and I feel less alone when awake, immersed in another country. Unfortunately I often find myself without sleep for thirty six hours and more, but I have learned to be flexible and take care of minor things like cooking dinner, grocery shopping, reading the newspapers and online news during such periods. I often think of how people take so much for granted, like being able to sleep at night.

But rather than the division of litigation with outraged patients on the one hand and physicians paying so much money for lawyers on the other, I would have liked the possibility of turning to the process of restorative justice like the Native Americans rather than retribution -- which is a conversation between the physician and myself that would have ended in peace and balance.

I am more than fortunate because my husband has always been by my side since he has been less burdened by his job, and is the one person who knows what I am going through. He drives me to all my doctors appointments because he understands how quickly I tire. My daughter Laurence sent me those puzzles immediately after my brain injury, and has kept reassuring me that brain cells keep growing and that having a new way of writing poetry is just a new normal. My granddaughter Ariel, sent me a teddy bear with the simple note "I love you." Such caring gestures filled me with joy and gratitude.

These illness and medical errors have taught me how to count my blessings and achievements despite their costs. After the brain injury, it took me six months just to write an article, something I used to write every day with great ease, but I had no intention of giving up my passion. My niece Michele who is more than busy as a professor and a writer has read all of my manuscripts since then. I am more than grateful for her time. But this problem has taught me that it is possible for light and darkness to be intertwined. I persisted and managed to write five books in the next seven years. I now refer to myself as a skinny tank always moving forward.

Coping with so many physical problems is also a blood wedding where I married the world. When I enjoyed good health I spent much of my time working for human rights, including five years working long hours with Lao refugees, but now I feel deeply connected to every single person who is struggling, and how we are all intertwined. As my life became a daily negotiation, I found myself reaching out to people who were in extremely difficult situations, including a Syrian refugee suffering from Post Traumatic Stress, and it was not difficult because I was able to share her feelings. To be able to share someone's pain instead of turning away is a healing act and I feel that we are here to make the world a better place by our actions. Although I used to do a great deal of volunteer work as well as my full time job, I still find many ways of reaching out, from helping a woman create a library she founded in Haiti, to teaching online courses in that university, to small things such as knitting scarves and afghans for the homeless.

Often people fear vulnerability, but everyone is vulnerable in some way. Then there is a quality that is often invisible and that is inner strength. A person such as myself, can be physically frail, but have great strength in reaching out to someone in need and accompanying them. Besides, giving of oneself is a source of joy. Reaching out to a small family, or to one person is a way of holding the earth in one's heart, of renewing the planet.

In his book *At the Will of the Body*, Arthur Frank makes the distinction between the word illness and disease, the latter referring to physiology, leaving out the fullness of a person's being. We speak of "falling ill," as if it were both an accident and a descent. I prefer to use the word "become," because it encompasses a much broader meaning and reverberates with possibilities. Similarly a person who suffers from cancer does not like to hear himself or herself described as "a cancer victim," or "a survivor," as if that phrase encompassed their entire identity.

I keep three cartoons of my favorite and more than witty cartoonist, Roz Chast who works for the New Yorker magazine and has published a wonderful book. They reveal people just sitting in front of a TV or sitting on a sofa with the comments, "Please don't get sick, I don't have the energy to deal with it right now," and "Thanks for not being under the weather, this is a very busy time for me" and finally "So glad you're in good health, it makes my life much easier." But these cartoons have had an unexpected sequel when President Donald Trump made fun of a disabled reporter.

Since the illnesses and malpractices I experienced, such as chronic insomnia, I found myself losing a number of friends since I could no longer share their activities, but also keeping a few meaningful relationships with people who understand who I really am. Over time I discovered that who I would become and what I would do with my life, would have to be spiritually meaningful. I found myself radically changing my values, seeking wisdom, understanding, and the enormity of kind gestures.

When I first became ill, I began reading widely in all religions especially Buddhist authors such as Sharon Salzburg, author of *A Heart as Wide as the World*. The works of Rebbe Nachman of Breslov or of the 13th century religious scholar and Sufi, mystic,

Rumi's poetry resonates with an understanding that radiates throughout my being. "Darkness is your candle./ Your boundaries are your quest./ You must have shadow and light source both./ Listen, and lay down your head under the tree of awe."[3]

As a poet, I had always been interested in Native American poets and now I turned to the great wisdom of these First Peoples. One of my favorite Native American poets, J.P. Dancing Bear, combines the voices of the earth with his love of Christ, revealing faiths that intertwine as do my own. A Navaho writer, Luci Tapahonso, also combined the two religions in her book that was partly written in the Dine (Navaho) language referring to celebrating Christmas as the luminaries, a road of lights.[4] She also reveals that prayers are part of the continuum of life. Native peoples including the Aztecs in Mexico intertwine Shaminsim and Christianity by worshiping our Lady of Guadelupe who appeared to Native Peoples that were caught between their culture and Western beliefs. What I also discovered through my ongoing reading is the vast inner space that I can tap into, serving as a counterpoint to my limited mobility and social space.

The noted Israeli poet Yehuda Amichai spoke ironically of the God zones in his area. Some people tend to tout their religions as if when we die there will be indeed separate places for their souls. Although religion often takes a political or ideological turn that has nothing to do with faith, we are here to respect and to rejoice in our diversity.

As always, I meditate every day lifting up my prayers for the world. Meditation has led me to the understanding that suffering is part of our human journey, and that it brings us not only compassion, but connection to everyone on this earth, from the women in the terrible Sudanese war who have been raped to the hungry children in Haiti. I no longer ask the question "Why me," but rather "Why not me." Through meditation, I have discovered that, although we cannot change our physical distress, we are always able to change our attitudes and thus acquire an inner peace and understanding.

Even though I have so little stamina, I am very much in the world. I have learned not to be drawn in by polemics. The pressures for visible success seem to be everywhere and, sometimes creep into our subconscious. I have always been fiercely independent, but the periods of quiet I have set aside help me to keep a distance from the messages that bombard us. As I continued my research and writing during the odd hours I have, sometimes writing in at 2:00 in the morning, my research became intertwined with my efforts to create change. I wrote books about people we marginalize; such as soldiers who return stateside with invisible wounds, women around the world who work for human rights in areas such as environmental racism. I did write a book, *Social Justice and the Power of Compassion* that includes a chapter on a foundation that brings together, Jews, Muslims and Christians around the world, but this essay is about my personal efforts.

One of those efforts is taking care of people who need help. They come from the Native American view of reciprocity, a sense of responsibility to one another and also of the concept of kinship. Native Americans' place a very high value on generations and family. However, their view of kinship also includes people who are not biologically related, a feeling I share. I have a long list of people whom I have loved and mothered, something that is very important to me and fills me with happiness.

For me the inner life is a sacred space and connecting to the lives people share with me is a web. This way of life is the one offered to us by Native American spiritual leaders who are known as "the Beloved Woman." Native Americans revere her. The role of older women as spiritual comes from the forebearers that too many of us are unaware of. Asudi, an elderly Cherokee has written, "Wisdom is with the aged, and understanding is in the length of days."[5]

Since my visit to Tahlequah decades ago, I have become enfolded in the Native American spirit, and work for balance, and also for diversity that honors minorities. I have come to understand how love and wisdom are the source of real power, not hierarchy, weapons, political status or great wealth. It's not that the latter ever mattered to me, but now I see them in a different way.

The Native Americans speak of the balance we need in our lives as strength and tenderness. Although I am physically frail, I have an inner strength and much compassion. And as Native Americans I feel that each moment when we reach out to help someone or to make peace has its own eternity. Also I know that as written in the Qur'an, saving one life is saving humanity, and I believe that there are no lesser or greater in this world of ours.

Patriarchy that streams through so many religions has not repressed the feminine spirit that is still with us. It holds the same view as our forebears, the Native Americans and Indigenous Peoples around the world, that the feminine spirit is concerned with interconnectedness and reveals the concept of balance that has been given to us by the First Peoples. In the words of the Cherokee writer, Awiakta "Grandmother Corn (Selu) is a mother, enabler, transformer, healer."[6]

In a society that measures so much by externals, it is comforting to remember that we all have a spiritual dimension that we can refer to in trying times, a life that can be as spacious as that of those who are able to travel great distances in their days. We can also reclaim our lives by continuing to give in different ways and by fashioning conversation so that we become present in people's consciousness and thus feel empowered.

Reverend Sam Oliver, a Spiritual Counselor for the Center for Hospice and Palliative Care in Cleveland, Ohio, wrote a book *Integrating the Feminine Spirit; Returning to the Womb of Creation*. He has written about the connection between soul and heart, and that by serving the needs of others "our hearts become synchronized with the pulse of Creation," an insight which has been given to us by the First Peoples from time immemorial.[7]

NOTES

1. Polk, Sam. "Wall Street Bro Talk." *International New York Times,* 7/10/2016.

2. Awiakta, Marilou. "Selu: Seeking the Corn Mother's Wisdom," Colorado: *Fulcrum Publishing*, 1993, 229.

3. Barks, C. with Moyne, J: "The Essential Rumi", San Francisco: *Harper*, 1996, 20. The quoted passages are from the poem *Enough Words?*

4. Tapahonso, Luci. "Blue Horses Rush In," *The University of Arizona Press*, 1996.

5. Awiakta, Marilou.

6. Ibid. p. 21.

7. Oliver, Sam. "Integrating the Feminine Spirit, Returning to the Womb of Creation," Bloomington, Indiana. *1stBooks-rev.* 2005, 68.

Acknowledgments

Maria Bernardi is the author of 12 non-fiction books, including *Mothers of Adult Children*, as well as eight poetry books, two of which have won awards. She is a former Professor of Political Science and Poetry workshops and a Visiting Scholar at the Environmental Studies Program at Brandeis University.

Pierre C. Bouvard is Chief Insights Officer for Cumulus Media and Westwood One where he develops media and marketing insights to support the firms 1100+ media sellers. Previously, Pierre was Senior Vice President of Sales for TIVO Research & Analytics and President of Sales for Arbitron Inc. Bouvard was also EVP at Coleman Insights, a leading radio industry market research and consulting firm. He regularly writes blogs for Everyone's Listening.

Christina Chiu is the author of a book of short stories, *Troublemaker and Other Saints*, as well as a novel. She is currently working on a memoir.

Tara Coyote has created a Wind Horse Sanctuary for people who are ill or grieving. She combines her background as a movement teacher with her experience as an Equine Facilitated learning instructor. The horses are a healing presence and the programs include the somatic experience of being present with one's body and emotions.

Wendy Devitt is the teacher of low vision students in grammar school. She volunteers by teaching Yoga to young students and teens. She is currently writing a memoir on her experience.

Nancy Gerber was a visiting lecturer in the English and Women's Studies departments of Rutgers-Newark. Currently she is an advanced candidate in psychoanalytic training at the Academy of Clinical and Applied , she is the author of two books: *Fire and Ice: Poetry and Prose* (Arseya, 2014), which was nominated for a Gradiva Award sponsored by the National Association for the Advancement of Psychoanalysis, and *Losing a Life: A Daughter's Memoir of Caregiving* (Hamilton, 2005), from which her essay was adapted.

Jean Gould is the editor of a number of books including *Seasons of Adventure; Traveling Tales and Outdoor Journeys of Women over 50* and *Hot Flashes From Abroad; Women's Travel Tales & Adventures*. She has written many articles and has traveled widely in Africa.

Preston Hood is the author of a poetry book *A Chill I Understand* and was the recipient of the Maine Literary Award for his poetry book *The Hallelujah of Listening*. Preston is widely published in numerous journals and anthologies. He is currently working on his memoir, and writing another book of poetry. He teaches Therapeutic Creative Writing & Integrative Restoration – IRest Yoga Nidra Meditation. He was featured in two films recently one about the PTSD of veterans and one of veterans reading their poems about their experience.

Victoria Molta is a writer whose work has appeared in numerous publications. As a person in recovery from mental health issues, her calling has been to immerse herself in the Connecticut mental health movement. For over thirty years, she has worked as an advocate and recovery support specialist.

Neil Ellis Orts is a writer and performer, living in Houston, Texas. His writing has appeared in literary journals, anthologies, and general interest magazines. His novella, *Cary and John,* was published in 2014.

Sister Pamela Smith, SS.C.M. is the author of twelve books on Biblical themes and environmental ethics. Books of meditations on the Holy Spirit, on grief, and a chapbook of poems and prose poems on living with diabetes are forthcoming from Twenty-Third Publications, ACTA Publications, and Finishing Line Press, respectively. She has been a teacher, principal, religious community and parish administrator, and currently serves as Secretary for Education and Faith Formation in the Catholic Diocese of Charleston.

Carol Van der Woude has written a number of articles on nursing, midwifery, home birth, and a novel, "Alisa's Letter: A Legacy of Faith," as a tribute to women that immigrated to Upper Michigan from Finland during the copper boom.

***